Don't Drop the Baby!

A New Dad's Guide to Keeping It Together

By Mark Hampton

A fun, loving, and humorous guide for new dads, packed with personal experiences, practical advice, and a whole lot of laughs. Because fatherhood is an adventure worth preparing for—with a smile.

Dedication

To my incredible wife, Monique. You took on pregnancy like a champion, and your strength during labor still amazes me. From the moment you became a mother, you've been nothing short of amazing. Your love, patience, and dedication have made our journey into parenthood an unforgettable one. I couldn't ask for a better partner.

To our son, Jameson, the most chilled, wonderful little guy anyone could ask for. You've made being a dad feel like the most natural, rewarding thing in the world. Thank you for making life so easy and filling our days with laughter and love.

Table of Contents

Introduction

Welcome, soon-to-be-dad (or maybe you're already in the thick of it, and if so, congratulations on finding time to read!). Whether you're freaking out a little—or a lot—about fatherhood, you're in the right place.

When I found out I was going to be a dad, it was during peak COVID, and let me tell you, the world was already upside down. Ultrasound appointments? Nope, I wasn't allowed in. I sat in the parking lot, waiting for updates over text, trying to piece together this life-changing moment through a phone screen. But, despite the challenges, one thing became clear: fatherhood was going to be one wild, unpredictable, and incredibly rewarding journey.

That's where this book comes in. **Don't Drop the Baby!** isn't your typical how-to guide for new dads. It's not here to overwhelm you with strict advice or a never-ending list of dos and don'ts. Instead, I want to offer something different—a funny, relatable, and reassuring look at what's ahead. After all, fatherhood isn't a straight path. It's full of diaper blowouts, coffee spills, sleepless nights, and moments so surreal and wonderful, you can't quite believe they're happening.

Through this book, you'll get practical advice, but I also hope to make you laugh and ease some of those jitters before the big day arrives (and oh boy, what a day it will be). You might find yourself nodding along, saying, "Yep, I'm already worried about that," or maybe you'll discover some things you didn't even think to worry about yet. Either way, we're going to tackle it all together—with humor, honesty, and a whole lot of patience.

From the moment you find out you're going to be a dad, everything changes. But that doesn't mean you have to lose your mind in the process. In fact, you're more prepared for this than you think. Trust me, if I can do it—spilled coffee, late car seat installation, and all—you can too.

So, grab a cup of coffee, take a deep breath, and let's get you ready for the ride of your life.

Welcome to fatherhood. You've got this. And if you don't, well, you will by the time you finish this book.

There's a moment in every man's life that fundamentally shifts his world—no, not when his favorite football team wins the championship or when he beats his personal best in the gym. I'm talking about the moment you find out you're going to be a dad. In that split second, when your partner looks at you with that mix of excitement, terror, and, possibly, nausea, your life as you knew it takes a sharp turn toward the wildest adventure yet.

For me, the moment didn't come as a surprise—my wife and I had planned to have a baby. It was something we both wanted, and like many couples, we expected it to be a journey full of those romantic, life-affirming milestones you see in movies. Spoiler alert: it wasn't. Not entirely, at least. When you're planning a baby in the middle of a global pandemic, let me tell you, the experience is slightly different than you might expect.

The Pregnancy Test: A Moment of Truth (and Panic)

So, there we were, deep in the stage of peak COVID-19, a time when hugging your neighbor was considered a felony, and toilet paper was more valuable than gold. We had our plan in place, our timelines set, and now, we just had to wait. When my wife took the pregnancy test, I was trying to stay calm. But any guy who tells you he was totally cool and collected while waiting for the results is either a liar or a robot.

When she came out holding the test, showing those magical two lines that confirmed the mission was a success, the world suddenly felt... different. I mean, sure, it was still a world where I had to wear a mask to take out the trash, but now, *I* was going to be a father. Cue every emotion possible hitting at once—excitement, fear, joy, uncertainty. It's like being on the highest rollercoaster drop, except you have no idea when (or if) you'll hit the bottom.

This is where the mind plays tricks on you. In the span of five minutes, I went from "I can totally handle this" to "How do you even hold a baby?" to "Am I mature enough for this?" to "Wait, does this mean I need a minivan?" Let me tell you, young dad-to-be, it's normal to feel a bit unhinged in those first moments.

First Reality Check: The Pandemic Parenting Paradox

As if learning to become a father wasn't daunting enough, the reality of COVID threw in some curveballs that I never saw coming. One of the toughest parts, which I hadn't anticipated, was the feeling of being disconnected from the process. You see, thanks to

COVID-19 restrictions, I wasn't allowed to attend any of the ultrasound appointments with my wife. That's right—the moments you imagine as being one of the most emotional, tear-jerking experiences as a dad-to-be were replaced by me sitting in the car, waiting for my wife to text me grainy images of the ultrasound.

Imagine this: you're sitting in a parking lot trying not to make eye contact with the equally anxious dude in the car next to you, and all you have is a phone in hand, waiting. When that first ultrasound picture came through, it was an overwhelming moment… in the sense that I had absolutely no idea what I was looking at. Was that a head? An arm? A futuristic blob from another dimension? I knew it was my kid, but the emotion was dulled by the fact that I wasn't physically there. COVID, man. It robbed me of the classic *dad-gets-emotional-over-the-first-ultrasound* moment.

And here's the thing: a lot of guys experienced the same thing during that time. It's not like in the movies where you're holding hands with your wife, watching in awe as the ultrasound tech points out all the little features. Nope. I got to experience it all via text messages, Zoom calls, and a few virtual high-fives. It felt weird, disconnected, and at times, a bit isolating. It wasn't nice for my wife either! The fact that she had to go through all her appointments alone, without her husband by her side, affected her in a way that left her feeling like a single mother during those visits. It certainly diffused the experience for the both of us, but we're now glad those restrictions have been terminated for everybody now.

If you're going through something similar, know that you're not alone, and those feelings of missing out are totally valid. What matters most is that you're there—emotionally, mentally—even if you can't physically be at every appointment. Don't let the circumstances dull the excitement. I had to learn that fatherhood isn't just about the big, cinematic moments; it's about showing up, even if that means through a screen at times.

What's Next? Preparing for Fatherhood Without Losing Your Cool

Let's be real: the moment you find out you're going to be a dad is quickly followed by the equally terrifying question of "What now?" Society tells you that you need to be prepared, but how do you prepare for something as unpredictable as raising a tiny human? Is there a manual? (Spoiler: not really.)

This is the point where every dad-to-be starts Googling like his life depends on it. Suddenly, you're reading about everything from the best cribs to what color baby poop is normal (yes, you'll find yourself having this conversation someday). It's like getting a crash course in survival, only the stakes feel impossibly high. So, here are some practical tips from a guy who's been there:

1. Embrace the Chaos

Fatherhood isn't a straight line; it's more like a squiggly one that loops back on itself, does a few cartwheels, and then leads you somewhere unexpected. And that's okay. Planning is good but understand that things rarely go according to the script. That doesn't mean you're doing it wrong; it means you're doing it *real*. Laugh at the chaos, because trust me, you're going to need a sense of humor.

2. The Nursery Trap

Ah yes, the nursery. The place where you'll be tempted to spend thousands of dollars on adorable but entirely unnecessary items. Let me save you some time and money: your baby doesn't care if their room is Pinterest-perfect. They don't even know they *have* a room. They'll be spending most of their time attached to you or in a crib, so as long as it's safe and comfy, you're golden. Pro tip: A diaper bin that actually seals in smells is worth its weight in gold.

3. Support Your Partner (and Don't Forget Yourself)

Being there for your partner during pregnancy is huge. She's going through some wild changes, and your role is to be the calm in the storm. Offer support, whether it's picking up the slack with housework or just being there to listen. That being said, don't forget to take care of yourself. Dads are often expected to be the strong, silent types, but this is a massive life change for you to. Find your own outlets, whether it's working out, talking to friends, or binge-watching dad videos on YouTube (I may or may not have done that last one).

The Emotional Rollercoaster: It's Okay to Be Scared

One of the things no one really tells you is that it's okay to be scared. I'll admit, when I found out I was going to be a dad, there were moments when I felt completely overwhelmed. I wasn't sure I was ready, I worried about the kind of dad I'd be, and I questioned if I'd be able to handle the responsibility.

Here's the thing: those fears are normal. Every new dad goes through them, whether they admit it or not. It's a big responsibility, and there's no perfect formula for success. But the fact that you care enough to worry is already a sign that you're going to be a great dad. Fatherhood is about showing up, being present, and learning as you go.

Your New Role: The Dad-to-Be Transformation

One of the strangest things that happens when you find out you're going to be a dad is how quickly you start to change. You're not just the guy who enjoys sports, binge-watches movies, or goes to the gym anymore—you're now on a path toward becoming "Dad."

It starts small. Maybe you find yourself lingering in the baby aisle at Target, or perhaps you're suddenly fascinated by strollers and car seats. (Trust me, the stroller decision is not to be taken lightly.) Before you know it, you're already thinking ahead—how you're going to teach your kid to ride a bike, how you'll coach their soccer team, or how you'll manage not to embarrass them in front of their friends.

But more than that, you begin to think about the kind of dad you want to be. And that's where the real growth happens. Because while fatherhood is full of hilarious moments and minor disasters, it's also about stepping up in ways you never knew you could. You're about to become someone's hero, and that's an amazing thing.

Conclusion: Welcome to the Dad Club

So, welcome to the Dad Club! It's a place full of high-fives, sleepless nights, and more baby wipes than you ever thought possible. It's a wild ride, but one worth taking. And if you're feeling nervous, scared, or unsure—that's normal. We've all been there. Fatherhood is a journey, and you're just getting started. Grab a coffee, find your sense of humor, and get ready for the adventure of a lifetime. You've got this.

Chapter 2

Surviving the Pregnancy Journey (Without Losing Your Mind)

Pregnancy. The magical, transformative experience where your partner grows an actual human-being inside of her. It's awe-inspiring, life-changing, and, let's be honest, sometimes completely bonkers. From the outside, it might seem like pregnancy is all glowing skin and cute baby bumps, but for dads-to-be, it's also a time of navigating unfamiliar terrain. You're stepping into new roles—supporter, cheerleader, snack-fetcher, and sometimes, the target of irrational frustrations. (And trust me, even if you think you know your partner, pregnancy has a way of introducing a few surprises.)

But before you panic, let's get one thing straight: you can do this. Whether you're an expectant father partnered with a pregnant woman or supporting her from the outside, your role is crucial. This chapter is about how to handle those nine months with humor, patience, and, most importantly, without losing your cool.

The Calm Before the Storm: First Trimester Reality Check

So, you've made it through the initial shock of finding out you're going to be a dad. Maybe the pregnancy was planned, like ours, or maybe it came as a complete surprise. Either way, you're in for an adventure. The first trimester is often referred to as the "calm before the storm," but it comes with its own set of challenges.

In my case, the early days of pregnancy were all about excitement and anticipation. We spent a lot of time talking about the future, what our baby might look like, and making lists of baby names (which, by the way, can turn into its own mini battle). But while we were excited, my wife also started feeling the early symptoms: fatigue, nausea, and the occasional mood swing.

Now, I have to say, I was pretty lucky. My wife was never the type to have those extreme pregnancy mood swings you see in the movies, where one minute she's laughing, and the next, she's throwing a plate across the room. However, that doesn't mean there weren't moments when emotions ran a little higher than usual. Hormones are no joke, and as a dad-to-be, your job is to weather those storms, even if they're just small gusts.

1. The "Why Are You Breathing So Loud?" Syndrome

There's a classic joke about pregnant women being annoyed by their partner's breathing, and as funny as it sounds, it's not entirely off the mark. During pregnancy, things that never bothered your partner before might suddenly become the most irritating things on the planet. For example, there were a few times when I could tell my wife was looking at me like, "If you chew that apple any louder, I might actually lose it."

It's important to remember that this isn't about you. Her body is going through a major transformation, and with that comes a lot of discomfort, both physically and emotionally. So, if you find yourself on the receiving end of some unexpected frustration, take a deep breath and let it go. You don't need to defend your apple-chewing technique.

2. How to Handle Mood Swings (and Keep Your Sanity)

Even if your partner isn't prone to massive mood swings, like mine, there will still be moments when the hormones kick in, and suddenly everything feels a little more intense. Here are a few tips for handling those moments:

- **Don't Take It Personally**: This is rule number one. If she's frustrated, moody, or emotional, it's not about you. It's about her body going through a major change. The best thing you can do is be patient, listen, and not escalate the situation.
- **Be Available Without Hovering**: One of the trickiest balances during pregnancy is being present and supportive without being overbearing. You don't need to solve every problem but being there to listen (even if she's venting about something that seems insignificant) is key. Sometimes, she just wants to be heard.
- **Laughter Is the Best Medicine**: Humor goes a long way in diffusing tension. If you can gently make her laugh during a tense moment, it can help shift the mood. Just make sure your jokes don't come off as dismissive—there's a fine line between being funny and being insensitive.
- **Create a Calming Environment**: Pregnancy can be stressful, and stress can exacerbate mood swings. Help create a calming environment by keeping things low-key when she's feeling overwhelmed. Whether that means running a bath, playing relaxing music, or just dimming the lights, small gestures can go a long way.

Getting Away: How We Survived by Taking Breaks (Joshua Tree, Anyone?)

When things started feeling a bit overwhelming, my wife and I found that taking short trips away from the usual day-to-day routine helped. One of the best trips we took during her pregnancy was to Joshua Tree National Park. Not only was it a chance to escape the stress of daily life, but it also gave us time to connect and just be together without the distractions of work, chores, or pregnancy planning.

Getting out in nature, especially in a place as surreal and beautiful as Joshua Tree, helped reset our minds. We spent our days hiking (well, light hiking—pregnancy limits your partner's stamina), enjoying the quiet desert, and having long conversations about what the future might hold. These kinds of trips don't have to be extravagant; they're just about finding space to breathe and reconnect.

Why Getting Away Helps

- **Stress Relief**: Pregnancy can feel overwhelming. Escaping to nature or even just going for a weekend getaway gives both of you a break from the routine and allows for relaxation.
- **Strengthening Your Bond**: Whether you're married, partners, or co-parents, this is a time to really strengthen your bond. Use trips or time away to focus on each other and the journey you're about to take as parents.
- **Perspective**: Sometimes, stepping away from the pregnancy planning and daily stress gives you a fresh perspective. For us, Joshua Tree became a place where we could talk about our hopes and fears for parenthood, all while surrounded by beautiful landscapes that reminded us how big the world is.

If a trip isn't possible, don't worry. Even something as simple as a day out in a nearby park, a drive in the countryside, or a mini staycation at home can provide the same benefits. The key is to find time to step out of the everyday stress and focus on your relationship.

Dealing with the "Pregnancy Brain" Phenomenon

Here's something you might not have anticipated: "pregnancy brain." It's a real thing. Your partner might forget things, misplace items, or suddenly stop mid-sentence and have no idea where she was going with her thought. It's not because she's suddenly lost all her mental faculties—it's because her brain is working overtime to grow a human. In short, give her a break.

For me, this phase wasn't so much frustrating as it was amusing. There were a few times when my wife would walk into a room with full confidence, ready to tackle something, only to stop and ask, "Why did I come in here again?" It happens.

How You Can Help with Pregnancy Brain

- **Be Patient**: If she forgets things, misplaces her keys for the third time that day, or can't remember the name of your best friend's dog, don't get frustrated. It's part of the process, and it's temporary.
- **Offer Gentle Reminders**: If she has an appointment, a work deadline, or something else important coming up, help her stay on track with gentle reminders. Just don't frame it as "You always forget," because that's not going to go over well.
- **Take on Mental Load**: This is a great time to step up and take on some of the mental load. Whether it's keeping track of bills, scheduling appointments, or organizing baby stuff, the less she has to worry about, the better.

Being There for Her (and Keeping Your Cool)

Pregnancy is a marathon, not a sprint. As the months go on, your partner is going to face more physical and emotional challenges, and your role is to be her support system. That means showing up in ways you might not have expected and learning to be adaptable. Here are a few key things to remember:

1. The Little Things Matter

It's easy to get caught up in the big stuff—doctor's appointments, baby gear, planning the nursery—but don't overlook the small, everyday gestures that show her you're there. Bringing her a snack when she's hungry, running a bath after a long day, or simply rubbing her back when she's uncomfortable goes a long way.

2. Listen (Even When It's Hard)

Pregnancy comes with a lot of emotions, and sometimes, your partner just needs to vent. You don't need to solve every problem she brings up; often, she just wants you to listen and validate her feelings. If she's frustrated, tired, or overwhelmed, let her talk it out without jumping into "fix it" mode.

3. Be Proactive, Not Reactive

Try to anticipate her needs before she has to ask. If she's craving something, offer to grab it for her. If she's mentioned being sore, offer a back rub before she asks. Being proactive shows that you're paying attention and that you're invested in making this process easier for her.

4. Take Care of Yourself, To

Supporting your partner through pregnancy is important, but don't forget to take care of yourself as well. It's easy to get so wrapped up in making sure she's okay that you neglect your own mental and physical health. But remember, this is a long journey, and you need to be at your best, too. Make time for things that help you recharge—whether that's hitting the gym, taking a walk, or even just having a quiet moment to yourself.

It's not selfish to take care of yourself. In fact, it's crucial. You can't be the best support for her if you're running on empty. So, make sure you're eating well, getting enough sleep (or as much as you can), and finding outlets for your stress.

Final Thoughts: The Dad-To-Be Survival Kit

Becoming a father starts long before your baby is born. The moment you find out you're expecting, you're already on the journey. Pregnancy is an emotional, physical, and mental rollercoaster for both of you, but it's also a time for growth—both as individuals and as a couple.

Here's a little recap of how to be there for her during pregnancy, whether you're the partner, co-parent, or a supporting figure:

- **Patience is your greatest tool**. Pregnancy is unpredictable, and emotions can run high. Stay calm, listen, and don't take things personally.
- **Find ways to de-stress together**. Whether it's a weekend getaway to Joshua Tree or just a long walk, find moments where you can reconnect and enjoy each other's company.
- **Handle mood swings with humor and understanding**. It's not about you, so don't get defensive. Instead, try to make her laugh or give her space when she needs it.
- **Take care of yourself**. You're both in this together, and that means you need to be in good shape mentally and physically to support her—and to prepare for the sleepless nights ahead!
- **Be proactive**. Anticipate her needs, offer help without being asked, and show her that you're in this together, every step of the way.
- **Don't forget to enjoy the ride**. Sure, pregnancy can be tough, but it's also an incredible time in your life. These are the months before you officially become a dad, so try to appreciate the small moments of joy, excitement, and even the funny mishaps along the way.

By keeping these things in mind, you'll not only survive the pregnancy journey, but you'll also strengthen your relationship and prepare yourself for the adventures of fatherhood ahead.

Becoming a new dad means stepping into the unfamiliar world of baby gear. Suddenly, you're bombarded with ads, lists, and well-meaning advice about gadgets, accessories, and products that claim to make your life easier. But how do you know which ones are useful, and which ones are just taking up space and draining your wallet? Let's break it down, so you don't end up with a garage full of untouched baby swings and redundant diaper warmers.

The Essentials: What You Actually Need

When it comes to baby gear, there's a fine line between practical and overkill. Here's a list of the tried-and-true essentials that will make your life easier as a new parent:

---

1. Car Seat (For Real This Time)

I get it—setting up the car seat feels like assembling a piece of IKEA furniture that holds the fate of the world. I put off installing mine until the last minute and ended up scrambling when my son arrived 8 days early. Don't make that mistake. *Pro tip*: Practice installing and uninstalling it before the big day arrives. The hospital won't let you leave without a properly installed car seat.

You don't need the most expensive car seat on the market, but make sure it's one that's safe, fits in your car, and is easy to click in and out. Trust me, when you're holding a crying newborn while trying to figure out how to secure the seatbelt, you'll thank yourself for getting a simple, user-friendly model.

---

2. A Good Stroller (That Fits Your Lifestyle)

Here's the thing about strollers: they come in all shapes, sizes, and price points. Some have enough cup holders and storage to make you feel like you're pushing a luxury SUV, while others are barely a step up from a shopping cart. You don't need to spend a fortune on a high-end model, but you do need something that matches your lifestyle.

If you're into walking or jogging, get one that's durable with decent wheels. If you're like me and live in a more urban area, a compact, lightweight stroller that's easy to fold and store is the way to go. But whatever you do, avoid strollers that need an engineering degree to collapse—they're fun in the showroom but a nightmare when you're wrestling with one hand and holding a baby in the other.

---

3. Diapers (Lots of Them)

This one's a no-brainer. Diapers are like oxygen—you don't realize how vital they are until you're out of them. I'd recommend stocking up on different sizes because babies grow fast. However, don't go overboard with newborn sizes, since your baby will outgrow them before you know it. Keep a healthy balance, and maybe even sign up for a subscription service to ensure you never have that *oh-no-we're-out-of-diapers* panic.

And no, you don't need the fanciest brand with all the extra padding and bells and whistles. Most diapers will get the job done just fine. Also, side note: expect your first attempt at changing one to be a comedic disaster. You're going to mess it up—probably more than once—but you'll get the hang of it.

---

4. A Baby Carrier

Having a good-quality baby carrier is life-changing. Whether you're going for a walk, doing some chores around the house, or even just trying to soothe a fussy baby, a carrier allows you to keep your hands free while still keeping your baby close. You'll want one that's comfortable for both you and the baby, adjustable, and easy to put on.

Carriers come in various styles, from wraps to structured designs. Honestly, the simpler, the better. Some of these things are like complicated jigsaw puzzles, and when your baby is screaming, you don't want to be fumbling around with 30 different straps. Find one that works, and you'll wonder how you ever lived without it.

---

5. A Simple, Safe Crib or Bassinet

Your baby needs somewhere safe to sleep (and by sleep, I mean nap sporadically while you hover nearby hoping for a miracle). You don't need a fancy, high-tech crib that monitors their every breath. A basic crib or bassinet that's up to safety standards will do the job just fine.

Pro tip: Skip the elaborate bedding and bumpers. They're not only unnecessary, but they can also pose safety risks. Keep it simple with a fitted sheet, and you're golden.

The Overhyped: What You Think You Need (But Definitely Don't)

Now, onto the fun part—the stuff that seems crucial, but you'll quickly realize is more trouble than it's worth.

1. Wipe Warmer

A wipe warmer sounds like a genius idea at first. After all, who wants to clean a baby's bottom with a cold wipe in the middle of the night? But trust me, babies don't care. The wipe warmer is one of those products that you'll use once or twice and then forget about entirely. Plus, warm wipes dry out faster, which means you're stuck with crusty wipes when you need them most.

2. Baby Food Makers

If you enjoy cooking, you might think a baby food maker is the way to go—just puree some veggies, and you've got healthy homemade meals for your little one. Here's the thing: you can do the exact same thing with a regular blender or food processor. Baby food makers are just expensive, miniaturized versions of appliances you probably already own. Save the counter space.

3. Designer Diaper Bags

Yes, diaper bags are essential—but do you really need one that costs as much as your first car? Functionality is way more important than brand names when it comes to diaper bags. You want a bag with lots of pockets, easy-to-clean material, and durability. Anything beyond that is just a flex you won't care about when you're digging through it in the middle of a public restroom.

4. Baby Shoes (Before They Can Walk)

Sure, tiny baby shoes are adorable. But unless your newborn is planning to walk down a runway (spoiler: they're not), shoes are a waste of money. They're difficult to keep on, babies grow out of them in a heartbeat, and your little one doesn't need them until they start walking. Stick with socks or soft booties and save the cute shoes for later.

5. Fancy Baby Clothes

It's hard to resist all those cute outfits at the store, but here's a reality check: babies outgrow clothes faster than you can change a diaper. Most of the time, your little one will be in comfortable onesies or sleepers. While a few nice outfits for photos or special occasions are fine, stocking up on expensive, fancy clothes is unnecessary. They'll probably wear that adorable outfit once before it's too small.

---

6. Bottle Sterilizers

While keeping your baby's bottles clean is important, you don't need a specialized machine to sterilize them. Boiling water or using a dishwasher with a sanitizing setting will do the trick just fine. The sterilizer just ends up taking up space and adding an extra step to an already busy routine.

Bonus: The "It's Up to You" List

There are some baby items that fall into a gray area—whether they're worth it or not depends entirely on your lifestyle and preferences.

---

1. Swings and Bouncers

Some babies love them, and others couldn't care less. If you find that your baby enjoys the movement, a swing or bouncer can be a lifesaver. But be aware that some of these contraptions are enormous and will take over your living room. If you decide to get one, keep the receipt just in case your baby isn't a fan.

---

2. Baby Monitor with All the Bells and Whistles

A baby monitor is definitely useful, but do you really need one with a night vision camera, temperature sensors, and two-way audio? Unless you're monitoring a space station, probably not. A basic video or audio monitor will work just fine and save you from obsessively checking a live feed.

---

3. Pacifiers

Some babies take to pacifiers like they've found their best friend; others want nothing to do with them. Keep a few on hand, but don't be surprised if your baby spits it out and gives you the side-eye.

Conclusion: Less Is More

When it comes to baby gear, less is more. Babies don't need all the latest gadgets and gizmos—what they need most is your love, attention, and care. Focus on the essentials that will make your life easier, and don't feel pressured to buy everything the baby registry checklist suggests. Parenthood is challenging enough without tripping over unnecessary baby gear in the middle of the night.

As with most things in fatherhood, the key is to adapt and figure out what works for you and your family. After all, no two babies are exactly alike—just like no two dads are, either. So, breathe easy, don't sweat the small stuff, and remember: no matter what gear you have or don't have, you've got this.

Chapter 4

The Day of The Birth – When It All Goes Down

The day your child is born will be one of the most incredible (and nerve-wracking) experiences of your life. Whether it happens early, on time, or fashionably late, there's nothing that fully prepares you for the moment when labor kicks in. You might have everything meticulously planned, down to the snacks in your hospital bag—or maybe you're more of the "wing it" type. Either way, it's going to be a whirlwind. And as the dad-to-be, your role on that day is essential.

Now, if you're like me, you'll think you're ready. Hospital bag? Packed. Snacks? Check. Car seat? Oh wait. About that… We'll get to my little oversight in a bit.

The point is, no matter how prepared you think you are, the day of the birth is unpredictable. And while your partner is doing all the hard work, there's plenty you can do to make things easier on her. Plus, a few laughs (even unintentional ones) can go a long way in keeping the mood light.

Getting the Call (Or the Nudge) – "It's Time!"

One minute, you're just living your normal life. The next, everything is about to change. Whether your partner's water breaks in the middle of the night, or she casually tells you, "I think it's happening," the rush of adrenaline is real. For me, that moment came eight days earlier than expected. I had everything ready to go, but the one thing I hadn't checked off the list was installing the car seat. Rookie mistake, right?

Of course, the fact that our son came early didn't leave me much room to defend myself. But let's be honest—even if he had been born on time, I probably still would've found a way to push it until the last minute. You live, you learn.

Lesson #1: Have the Car Seat Ready

Seriously, don't make my mistake. Install that car seat *now*. Not tomorrow, not the day after. Do it now. You might think, "I have plenty of time," but babies are on their own schedule. The last thing you want to be doing when you're supposed to be rushing to the hospital is fumbling with straps and buckles while trying to watch YouTube tutorials on car seat installation.

The Hospital Dash – Stay Cool, Dad

Once labor starts, everything seems to go into fast forward. You've packed the bags (or at least you think you have), and now it's time to get to the hospital. Depending on where you live, this part could be a leisurely drive or an all-out race against traffic. Either way, try to stay calm. Your partner needs you to be focused and composed. You don't want to be that dad who shows up to the hospital out of breath, sweating, and panicking. Keep your cool. If you can.

I remember driving to the hospital, trying to be as calm as possible. My wife was in early labor, and we both knew it could be a long day (and night). But no matter how much you've heard about labor being long, nothing quite prepares you for how time will start to feel. At first, it's slow, then suddenly, you blink, and you're in hour 18 wondering how the sun is setting again.

Labor – The Waiting Game

Labor is different for every woman. Some labors are quick, others are long (like our 23-hour marathon). And while the moms are the ones doing all the hard work, dads, you're going to be in it for the long haul too. Your main job is to support her, make sure she's as comfortable as possible, and keep the mood light if you can.

1. Be the Calm in the Storm

There's a lot going on during labor. Nurses coming in and out, doctors checking in, beeping monitors, and your partner working through contractions. It can feel a bit overwhelming, especially if it's your first time. But as the dad, your role is to be the calm in the storm. You're her anchor, the steady hand in the chaos. Even if inside, you're freaking out a little bit, try to keep a cool exterior.

2. Timing Contractions Like A Pro

One of the first tasks you'll probably be given is timing contractions. Trust me, this will make you feel like you're contributing something meaningful. Download an app (there are tons) and start timing. Even though it can feel repetitive, it helps keep you focused and gives your partner a sense of progress. Plus, it's a nice way to feel involved when most of the labor process is out of your hands.

3. Snacks and Comforts

Labor can be long, and no one does well on an empty stomach. Make sure you have snacks on hand—not just for her, but for you, too. And while it's tempting to sneak a bite when she's resting, be mindful that hospital rooms can be small, and the smell of certain foods can be less than pleasant during labor.

Also, pack little things that might make the experience more comfortable for her. Pillows from home, lip balm, a playlist of her favorite songs—these small comforts can make a big difference in her mood.

The Coffee Incident – Laughing Through the Pain

Now, speaking of snacks and drinks, let me share one of the lighter moments from our labor experience. It was around hour 15 or so, and I was doing my best to stay awake and alert. So, naturally, I turned to coffee. While my wife was lying there, breathing through contractions, I took a sip of coffee to keep myself going.

But, in one of those moments where life decides to remind you that you're not in control, I somehow managed to spit that coffee right out of my mouth and all over her. Yep. While she's in pain, suffering through contractions, I accidentally sprayed her with hot coffee. It wasn't one of my finer moments, but to this day, it's something we still laugh about.

Lesson #2: Maybe Skip the Coffee (or at Least Be Careful)

If you're going to drink coffee or eat anything while your partner is in labor, do it with caution. You're already on thin ice because she's the one doing the hard work, and if you mess up like I did, you're not going to hear the end of it. Thankfully, my wife has a great sense of humor, and we both laughed it off. But it could have gone another way…

Supporting Her Through the Pain

Labor pain is no joke. Watching someone you love go through intense contractions and discomfort can be tough. You want to do everything you can to help, but sometimes there's not much you can do besides being present. That said, there *are* a few things you can do to make her more comfortable.

1. Be Her Advocate

Hospitals can be intimidating places, especially when you're dealing with doctors and nurses who are busy with other patients. One of your most important roles is to be your partner's advocate. If she's too tired or in too much pain to speak up, it's your job to make sure her needs are being met. Whether it's asking for more pain relief options, a different position, or just more time with the doctor, don't be afraid to speak up on her behalf.

2. Know When to Be Quiet

This one's important. There are going to be moments when your partner needs quiet and focus, and there are going to be moments when she wants you to hold her hand and offer words of encouragement. The trick is knowing when to do which. If she's going through a particularly intense contraction, it's not the time for you to start telling her about the latest sports scores. Read the room. Silence can be golden during labor.

3. Help Her with Breathing

If you've been to any prenatal classes, you'll know that breathing techniques are a big part of managing labor pain. Be ready to help your partner through her breathing exercises, even if you both feel a little silly doing it. It might not seem like much but reminding her to breathe through the contractions can really help.

4. Keep the Energy Positive

Labor can be exhausting, and it's easy for the energy in the room to start feeling heavy, especially as the hours tick by. Your job is to keep things positive without being overly chipper (because no one likes the guy who's too happy when everyone else is exhausted). Offer encouragement, remind her how amazing she's doing, and keep things light when you can. A little laughter can go a long way.

The Home Stretch – Pushing and the Big Moment

After hours of labor, the moment finally comes. The pushing phase. This is where things get real. For some women, this part lasts a few minutes; for others, it can take hours. Either way, this is when your partner will need you the most.

1. Be Her Cheerleader

During pushing, your partner is going to need all the encouragement she can get. Cheer her on, remind her how strong she is, and tell her how close she is to meeting your baby. It's a grueling process, but your words can make all the difference.

2. Don't Forget to Breathe Yourself

This moment is intense. Emotions are running high, and it can feel like the room is buzzing with energy. Make sure you're taking deep breaths too and staying focused. You don't want to be the dad who passes out in the delivery room (yes, it happens).

3. Be Ready for Anything

Birth is unpredictable. No matter how much you plan or prepare, things might not go exactly as you imagined. Maybe you were hoping for a natural birth, but a C-section becomes necessary. Maybe you had a birth playlist ready to go, but things are happening too fast for any of that. The best thing you can do is stay flexible, roll with the punches, and be ready for anything.

For example, when our labor hit the 20-hour mark, we were beyond exhausted. It felt like time was standing still, and everything we had prepped for seemed to go out the window. But one thing I learned is that you've got to just be present in the moment. The plans you made are just guidelines. The real goal is to get through it together, and most importantly, to safely welcome your little one into the world.

That First Cry – Welcome to Fatherhood

And then, after hours of hard work, pushing, and emotions running high, you'll hear it. That first cry. It's a sound that will change your life forever. In that instant, all the waiting, all the nerves, and all the stress disappear, replaced by awe and an overwhelming sense of love. You're a dad now.

I'll never forget hearing my son's first cry after those long 23 hours of labor. It was surreal. It didn't matter that I was tired or that we'd been through such a long process. In that moment, nothing else existed except for him. My son. That's the moment it all feels real, and trust me, the emotions will hit you like a freight train.

Lesson #3: Let Yourself Feel Everything

It's okay to get emotional. In fact, it's nearly impossible not to. Don't feel like you have to be the "tough guy" or hold back the tears. The birth of your child is one of the most emotional experiences you'll ever have. Embrace it. Let yourself feel the joy, the relief, and the overwhelming love that comes with that first cry.

What You Can Do in the Delivery Room

The delivery room is a whirlwind of activity, and while the doctors and nurses are focusing on your partner, you might feel a bit like a spare part. But trust me, you're an essential part of the team. Here's how you can stay involved and helpful:

1. Be the Go-To Person for Questions

During labor and delivery, your partner might not be in the best position to answer questions or make decisions. That's where you come in. Doctors and nurses might ask about pain relief options, positioning, or next steps. Make sure you know your partner's wishes ahead of time so you can step in and be her voice if she's too tired or focused to speak up.

2. Capture the Moment (When Appropriate)

Some couples want photos or videos of the birth. If that's something you and your partner agreed on, it's your job to play photographer. But don't get so wrapped up in trying to capture the moment that you forget to experience it. Take a few pictures if that's your plan, but be present for the actual birth. There's no do-over for this moment.

3. Cut the Cord (If You Want To)

This one's optional, but many dads are given the opportunity to cut the umbilical cord. It's a symbolic and emotional gesture—one that marks the beginning of your journey as a father. If you're up for it, go ahead and do it. But if the idea of handling sharp scissors in a high-pressure moment doesn't appeal to you, don't worry about it. There's no right or wrong decision here.

Post-Birth Chaos and Relief

Once the baby is born, the atmosphere in the room changes almost instantly. The focus shifts from labor to making sure the baby is healthy and that mom is okay. The room that was once filled with tension and pain is now filled with joy, exhaustion, and a sense of relief.

1. Stay Close to Your Partner

After all that hard work, your partner is going to need you more than ever. She's just been through an incredible (and likely exhausting) experience, and she'll appreciate having you by her side. Hold her hand, tell her how amazing she did, and share that first precious moment with your newborn together.

2. Skin-to-Skin Contact

If possible, take part in skin-to-skin contact with your baby. This isn't just something for moms—dads can benefit from it too. Holding your baby against your bare chest helps with bonding and can be incredibly soothing for both of you. Plus, there's nothing quite like that first time you hold your child in your arms.

The Car Seat Moment – Reality Check

So, let's circle back to the car seat. After all the excitement of birth, when it's finally time to go home, you'll be hit with the reality that you're now responsible for a tiny human. And in my case, that reality smacked me in the face when I realized we didn't have the car seat set up.

Luckily, the hospital staff were very understanding (and not at all surprised), and after a bit of fumbling and adjusting, we got it installed. But trust me when I say this: don't be like me. Get the car seat installed *before* labor starts, no matter how far off the due date seems.

The Ride Home – The Real Adventure Begins

That first drive home is surreal. You'll probably be driving at 10 mph, terrified of every bump in the road, with one eye glued to the rearview mirror checking on the baby. Welcome to fatherhood. It's a ride that's as thrilling as it is terrifying, and it starts the moment you leave the hospital.

But as nerve-wracking as it might be, remember that you're now equipped with something far more powerful than any amount of preparation: love. You've got this. Whether you're the guy who forgot the car seat or the dad who accidentally sprayed his wife with coffee during contractions, you'll figure it out. And those little mishaps? They'll be the stories you laugh about for years to come.

Final Thoughts: You're Ready, Even If You Don't Feel Like It

If there's one thing I want you to take away from this chapter, it's that no matter how unprepared or nervous you might feel, you're ready for this. Being a dad isn't about being perfect or having all the answers. It's about showing up, being there for your partner, and embracing every chaotic, beautiful moment that comes your way.

Birth day is just the beginning. The real adventure starts the moment you hold that tiny baby in your arms, and trust me, it's going to be the ride of your life.

So, you've made it through the labor. Congrats! You've experienced the emotional rollercoaster of seeing your baby for the first time, you survived the car ride home (hopefully with the car seat securely in place), and you're finally settling into the reality of being a dad. And then… it hits you. Well, not *you*, but something else. That first diaper change.

I'm going to be brutally honest here: changing diapers is one of those things no one is ever truly prepared for. You can watch a thousand YouTube tutorials, listen to your friends' horror stories, and read every baby book on the shelf, but until you're there, knee-deep in diaper duty, nothing really prepares you for the true art of *dealing with poop*.

I'd never changed a diaper before, so when it was my turn to dive in, I thought, "How hard can it be?" Spoiler alert: fairly hard. What I thought was going to be a simple swap of a dirty diaper for a clean one turned into a scene from a bad comedy sketch.

But before we dive too deep into my personal diaper-changing debacles, let's talk about the basics—because every new dad needs to know the ropes.

The First Diaper: Brace Yourself

Changing diapers is a rite of passage for all new dads, and nothing quite prepares you for the first one. The first diaper is not like the regular diapers you'll face later on. Nope. It's something called *meconium*. Sounds like a science-fiction material, right? Well, let me tell you, it looks like something straight out of a sci-fi horror movie. It's thick, tar-like, and you'll wonder if your child somehow swallowed crude oil in utero.

When I first encountered meconium, I had a moment of sheer disbelief. "Is this normal? Should I call a doctor?" But fear not—meconium is perfectly normal. Your baby's digestive system is just clearing out all the stuff they were storing up before birth. It's gross, yes, but thankfully, it only lasts for the first few days.

Lesson #1: Preparation is Key

Let's rewind to my first attempt at diaper changing. I had no idea what I was doing, but I was armed with confidence (and a pack of baby wipes). That's all you need, right? Wrong. What you need, first and foremost, is a **plan**.

Here's what I learned through trial and (a lot of) error:

1. **Gather Everything You Need First.** Don't start the change and then realize halfway through that you forgot the wipes, a fresh diaper, or a changing mat. Babies are quick, and they're escape artists. One second, you're holding their legs up, the next second, they've kicked themselves free, and chaos ensues.
2. **Use More Wipes Than You Think You Need.** One wipe is never enough. Two wipes? Maybe. Three wipes? Now we're talking. You're going to want to be thorough because there's nothing worse than thinking you're done, only to realize… you're not.
3. **Expect the Unexpected.** Babies have this magical ability to time their bodily functions with pinpoint accuracy. You'll think you're done; you'll be in the middle of fastening that fresh, clean diaper, and suddenly… they go again. Right there. It's like they're testing you, daring you to quit. Don't. You're in this for the long haul.

The Diaper Changing Battlefield

When you're first learning how to change diapers, it feels a bit like you're gearing up for battle. You're entering unknown territory, and your opponent—small though they may be—is cunning. They can strike at any moment, and usually, it's when you least expect it.

Let me paint you a picture of my first diaper-changing disaster. I had my son on the changing table, and everything seemed to be going well. I got the old diaper off, wiped him clean, and just as I reached for the new diaper… boom! He decided that was the perfect moment to "go" again. And not just a little. No, this was an all-out assault. I panicked, fumbled for more wipes, but by then, it was too late. The damage was done. Poop was *everywhere*.

This, my fellow dads, is the reality of diaper duty. It's messy, it's unpredictable, and sometimes, you just have to laugh through it. Because if you don't, you might cry.

Lesson #2: The Art of the Quick Change

Now that you're mentally prepared for the messiness, let's talk strategy. Diaper changing is all about speed, efficiency, and staying calm under pressure. Here are a few pro tips I've picked up along the way:

1. **Speed is Your Friend.** The quicker you can get the old diaper off and the new one on, the better. Babies don't like being exposed to the cold air, and they'll let you know it. Plus, the longer they're "free," the more likely they are to have an accident. So, practice your quick-change skills. The goal is to be as fast as possible without sacrificing cleanliness.
2. **Distract the Baby.** Babies are squirmy, especially as they get older. To keep them still while you're changing the diaper, try giving them a toy or talking to them in a

silly voice. Anything to keep their little hands (and feet) occupied while you're doing the dirty work.

3. **Double Check Everything.** Before you declare the diaper change a success, double-check your work. Make sure the diaper is snug, but not too tight, and that there are no gaps where leaks could happen. Because leaks will happen, and trust me, you don't want to deal with the aftermath of a diaper blowout.

The Diaper Blowout – Every Parent's Nightmare

Speaking of blowouts, let's talk about them. Every parent experiences at least one major diaper blowout, and if you're lucky, it'll happen when you're at home. If you're not so lucky, it'll happen when you're out in public, surrounded by people, with no backup clothes in sight. Been there, done that.

A diaper blowout is when the diaper simply cannot contain what's inside, and it *escapes*. It can be up the back, down the legs, or both. There's no predicting when or where it'll happen, but when it does, you'll know. The first time it happened to me, we were at the park. I picked my son up out of his stroller, and suddenly, I felt something warm on my arm. Yep. Blowout. And we were *miles* from home.

Lesson #3: Always Have a Backup Plan

If there's one piece of advice I can give you as a dad, it's this: **always** have a backup plan. Whether you're at home or out and about, always have extra diapers, wipes, and a change of clothes on hand. You never know when disaster is going to strike, and the last thing you want is to be caught unprepared in a public place with no clean clothes for the baby (or yourself).

Nighttime Diaper Changes: A Special Kind of Torture

Now, let's talk about nighttime diaper changes. These are a special kind of torture, and if you're lucky, your baby will eventually sleep through the night without needing one. But in the early days, nighttime changes are unavoidable.

You'll be half-asleep, fumbling with the diaper in the dark, trying not to wake the baby any more than necessary. The key here is to be *as quick and quiet as possible*. Keep the lights low, use a gentle voice, and pray that your baby falls back to sleep afterward. Spoiler: they probably won't.

One of my first nighttime changes was a disaster. I was trying to be quiet, but in my sleepy haze, I dropped the wipes container. The loud *thud* woke both my wife and the baby, and suddenly, instead of a quick change, we were all wide awake and dealing with a crying infant. Lesson learned: get everything you need in place *before* you start the change.

The Rookie Mistakes Every Dad Makes

We've all been there—rookie mistakes are part of the learning process. Here are a few common ones I've made (and you probably will too):

1. **Putting the Diaper on Backwards.** Yep, I did that. It wasn't until I tried to fasten the tabs and realized something was wrong that I figured it out. The front is where the pictures are, folks. Remember that.
2. **Not Fastening the Diaper Tight Enough.** I thought I was being kind by leaving the diaper a little loose, but all that did was cause leaks. Tighten it up! You want that thing snug.
3. **Underestimating the Pee Fountain.** Ah yes, the famous pee fountain. If you have a baby boy, you'll quickly learn that the moment you take off the diaper, there's a high chance you'll be sprayed. Cover that thing up with a wipe or a towel, or you'll find yourself drenched.

Final Thoughts: It's Not Glamorous, But It's Love

At the end of the day, diaper duty isn't glamorous. It's messy, it's exhausting, and it's sometimes downright disgusting. But here's the thing: it's also one of the most intimate, loving things you'll do as a dad. Taking care of your baby's needs, even the gross ones, is a way of showing love. It's part of the package deal, and after a while, you won't even flinch at the sight of a dirty diaper.

So, embrace it. Laugh at the mishaps, roll with the messes, and know that every diaper you change is another small victory in the wild adventure of fatherhood.

Chapter 6

Paternity Leave – The Hidden Benefits of Late-Night Shifts

Ah, paternity leave. It's the moment you've been waiting for—your chance to take a break from work, bond with your baby, and help your partner navigate those early days of parenthood. Or so you thought. In reality, paternity leave is a rollercoaster of sleepless nights, diaper changes, and figuring out how to function on minimal sleep. But here's the twist: if you're like me and you've worked nights before, you might actually find yourself a bit ahead of the game.

When my son was born, I was used to getting up early (or rather, staying up late and waking up early, thanks to my night shifts). This turned out to be a hidden advantage. While many new dads are struggling with the abrupt shift in their sleep patterns, I felt somewhat okay. I was already accustomed to the whole "sleep when you can" mentality. But even with my night owl habits, paternity leave was still an adventure filled with surprises.

Let's dive into what you can expect during paternity leave, especially if you've never had the pleasure of handling a newborn's schedule. I promise to keep it funny, insightful, and as real as possible.

The New Dad Schedule – Or Lack Thereof

First things first: there is no set schedule with a newborn. Forget about your well-ordered life and embrace the chaos. Babies have their own internal clocks, and they're not exactly synchronized with yours. My son's schedule seemed to revolve around eating every two hours, sleeping for short bursts, and keeping us on our toes.

One of the most significant adjustments for me was the new "schedule." As a night worker, I was used to being up at odd hours, but this was a whole new ball game. Our baby's feeding and sleeping patterns had no regard for normal human schedules. It was like trying to work out a system for an alien life form.

Here's what a typical day (or rather, a typical set of hours) might look like:

1. **Midnight Feeding:** Just as you're getting comfortable in bed, your baby decides it's time for a midnight snack. You stumble out of bed, half-asleep, and fumble with the bottle or your partner's breast (if breastfeeding). This might involve a bit of crying, some burping, and a lot of bleary-eyed confusion.
2. **Early Morning Cry:** After you've just managed to get the baby back to sleep, they're up again, and this time it's an early morning cry. The cycle repeats. You begin to understand the true meaning of sleep deprivation.

3. **Daytime Nap Time:** If you're lucky, you might get a chance to nap when the baby does. If not, you're in for a long day of trying to stay awake and be a functional human being. This is where having night shift experience comes in handy. While most people struggle to stay awake during the day, I found myself a bit more adaptable to the erratic sleep patterns.

The First Week: Survival Mode

The first week of paternity leave is like being thrown into survival mode. You're figuring out the basics of baby care, learning how to manage on minimal sleep, and trying to be supportive to your partner.

During that week, everything felt like a blur. I remember one day; my wife and I were trying to get our son to nap. He was crying, we were exhausted, and we had just about given up hope of finding any quiet. I attempted to soothe him by singing lullabies. Now, I'm no singer, but I gave it my all. Our son, being the tough critic that he is, cried even harder. I took that as a sign to stick to my day job—whatever that is now.

Lesson #1: Embrace the Chaos

One of the most important lessons I learned during paternity leave is to **embrace the chaos**. Things will not go according to plan, and that's okay. Your baby doesn't care about your schedule, your to-do list, or your need for a full night's sleep. They're living in their own little world, and you're just along for the ride.

Instead of stressing about the lack of routine, focus on making the best of each moment. Laugh at the little mishaps, like the time you accidentally put the diaper on backwards (again) or the time you forgot to add formula to the bottle. These moments are part of the adventure, and they'll make for great stories later on.

The Sleep-Deprived Dad: Functioning on Empty

Sleep deprivation is a real challenge, but if you're used to working nights, you might handle it better than most. My previous experience with night shifts meant I was already accustomed to functioning on limited sleep. While I still had my fair share of sleep-deprived moments, I found myself more resilient to the erratic sleep patterns of parenthood.

But let's be honest—no amount of night-shift experience can fully prepare you for the exhaustion of new parenthood. There will be moments when you're so tired you start talking to the baby in gibberish or try to make coffee with baby formula. It's all part of the fun.

One trick I learned was to find small moments of rest when I could. If the baby napped, I napped. If my wife took over for a while, I took the opportunity to close my eyes for a bit. Every little bit of sleep helps, and it's important to take care of yourself so you can take care of your family.

Supporting Your Partner: Teamwork Makes the Dream Work

During paternity leave, it's crucial to remember that you're a team with your partner. You're both navigating this new territory together and supporting each other is key. Here's how you can be the best teammate:

1. **Share the Load:** If you're both awake during a nighttime feeding or diaper change, take turns. This way, neither of you is left feeling completely exhausted. Share responsibilities and communicate about what needs to be done.
2. **Be Understanding:** Your partner is likely going through her own challenges with postpartum recovery, sleep deprivation, and adjusting to motherhood. Be patient, offer support, and recognize that you're both in this together.
3. **Celebrate the Small Wins:** Take time to acknowledge and celebrate the little victories. Whether it's successfully getting the baby to sleep for a few hours or just managing to get through the day without losing your mind, every win is worth celebrating.

The Joys of Bonding Time

One of the hidden gems of paternity leave is the opportunity to bond with your baby. You'll be amazed at how quickly you can form a strong connection during those early days. Whether it's feeding, changing diapers, or just spending time together, each moment is an opportunity to build a relationship with your little one.

For me, some of the most memorable moments were the quiet times I spent with my son. There was something incredibly peaceful about holding him and watching him sleep, knowing that I was his whole world. These moments made all the sleepless nights and chaotic days' worth it.

The New Dad Realizations

Paternity leave is a time of significant change, and with that change come new realizations. Here are a few things I learned during my time off:

1. **You're More Resilient Than You Think:** The exhaustion, the mess, and the constant demands of parenthood can be overwhelming, but you're more capable than you realize. You'll surprise yourself with how well you can handle it all.
2. **You'll Discover New Skills:** Diaper changing, bottle feeding, and soothing a crying baby—these are skills you didn't know you had until you were thrust into the role. Embrace the learning curve and enjoy the process of discovering what you're capable of.
3. **The Little Things Matter:** It's easy to get caught up in the big challenges of parenthood, but don't forget to appreciate the small moments. The smiles, the coos, and the tiny milestones are what make it all worth it.

The Return to Work: A New Chapter

As paternity leave comes to an end, you'll face the transition back to work. It's a mixed bag of emotions—excitement about returning to your routine and sadness about leaving your baby. It's normal to feel conflicted but remember that your role as a dad doesn't end when you go back to work. The skills and experiences you gained during paternity leave will stay with you, and you'll continue to be an essential part of your child's life.

One piece of advice for the transition back to work: **keep the lines of communication open** with your partner. The changes you've experienced as a family will continue, and working together to navigate this new phase will help you both adjust more smoothly.

Final Thoughts: Embracing the Chaos and Finding Joy

Paternity leave is an incredible opportunity to bond with your baby, support your partner, and adjust to the new dynamics of parenthood. It's a time of chaos, sleep deprivation, and unexpected challenges, but it's also a time of profound joy and connection. Embrace the messiness, laugh through the challenges, and savor every moment with your little one.

As you navigate this new chapter, remember that you're not alone. Every new dad goes through the same trials and triumphs, and together, you'll find your way. Enjoy the journey, cherish the memories, and know that every moment, no matter how difficult, is part of the beautiful adventure of fatherhood.

So, here's to you, new dad. You've got this. And if you can survive the diaper duty and sleepless nights, you can handle anything that comes your way.

Chapter 7

Mastering the Night Shift—Surviving Those Sleepless Nights

Welcome, brave fathers, to the battle that no amount of preparation can truly equip you for: the night shift. Those magical hours between sunset and sunrise, where the world falls into peaceful slumber—except, of course, for you, your partner, and your newborn baby, who seems to think the middle of the night is the perfect time to party. If you haven't already figured it out, newborns are nocturnal creatures, programmed to wake you up just as you've drifted off.

The truth is those early days with your baby are as much a mental endurance test as they are a crash course in survival. As a dad, you'll learn that nighttime is when the real challenges happen. But fear not, young father, for with the right strategy (and maybe a strong cup of coffee), you'll emerge victorious. And if nothing else, you'll at least survive.

Let's dive into the chaos of the night shift—complete with a few tips, tricks, and humorous observations to get you through it.

The Nighttime Routine: When Sleep Becomes a Fantasy

Here's the thing no one tells you: once your baby arrives, you'll enter a state of permanent sleep deprivation. You'll forget what uninterrupted sleep feels like, and you'll cherish even the briefest of naps. But before you panic, know that it's survivable. You just need to adjust your expectations and get into a rhythm that works for everyone.

In our case, my wife and I knew early on that teamwork was key. She breastfed, so when the baby woke up in the middle of the night, I'd handle the diaper change and then hand our son over to her for feeding. This system allowed us to divide the duties and ensured that one of us wasn't running on empty while the other snoozed away. Did it always go smoothly? Absolutely not. But having a plan in place made those late-night wakeups a little more bearable.

Surviving the Night Shift: Tips for Getting Through It

Since you're not a robot, sleep is a necessity, not a luxury. The trick to surviving the night shift as a dad is to embrace the chaos, laugh at the absurdity, and adopt a few practical strategies to make it through the dark hours. Here's what worked for us—and what might help you, too.

---

1. Teamwork Makes the Dream Work

Whether you're handling this whole parenting thing solo or working alongside a partner, the golden rule is **you're in this together**. There's no room for one person to shoulder all the responsibility while the other peacefully sleeps through the night. Establish a system that works for both of you. Maybe you take turns, swapping responsibilities each night, or maybe you divide duties like we did—one person handles the diaper, the other handles the feeding.

My wife and I had a pretty solid routine going after a while. We'd rotate well and, importantly, communicate. There were moments when she needed more rest, and I'd take over for longer stretches. Other nights, I was the one who needed an extra hour of sleep, and she graciously stepped up. When you're exhausted and bleary-eyed, it's easy to get snappy or frustrated, but it's crucial to remember you're both struggling. The key is empathy and understanding that your partner's exhaustion is as valid as yours. And yes, this means there's no "keeping score" about who got more sleep.

---

2. Communication is Key

This might sound like basic advice, but during the haze of sleep deprivation, communication becomes both more challenging and more important. You'll be tempted to assume the other person knows what you're thinking or feeling but trust me—they don't. Talk about your needs and how you're feeling. If you're overwhelmed, speak up. If you need a break, ask for it. And, equally important, listen when your partner does the same.

I'll be honest—there were nights when the lack of sleep made us both cranky. On more than one occasion, I made the rookie mistake of thinking I could handle it all without asking for help. Spoiler: this doesn't work. It's okay to admit you're tired or that you need a break. It doesn't make you any less of a dad or a partner. The sooner you communicate openly with each other, the easier the night shift becomes.

---

3. Master the Art of the Power Nap

During the night shift, you won't be getting those luxurious eight hours of sleep. You'll be lucky if you string together four hours, let alone two. The secret to survival? Power naps. Learn to fall asleep quickly and get in those precious 20-30 minutes whenever you can. Don't waste time scrolling through your phone—just close your eyes and drift off as soon as your baby does.

As I worked nights before becoming a dad, I thought I'd have the upper hand when it came to functioning on little sleep. Let me tell you, nothing can prepare you for the type of exhaustion a newborn brings. But those 20-minute naps were lifesavers. As soon as our son fell asleep after a feeding, I'd crash on the couch for a bit. It wasn't much, but it was enough to keep me going.

4. Technology is Your Friend (Sometimes)

There's no shame in using a little tech to make the night shift easier. White noise machines, baby monitors with night vision, apps that track feeding times—use them all if you feel like you do need additional help. Anything that helps you keep track of your baby's schedule or makes it easier to fall back asleep is a win.

We became huge fans of our baby scheduling app. Well, for me it was highly useful because it allowed me to be on top of things, especially when my wife returned to work, and I was home with my son during the day. And the white noise machine? That thing was a godsend, for both the baby and for us. If you haven't yet invested in some helpful gadgets, now's the time to do it.

5. Expect the Unexpected

Babies don't follow schedules, no matter how much you want them to. You might think you have things under control one night, only for your baby to decide to throw a curveball the next. Expecting the unexpected is half the battle. Stay flexible, go with the flow, and try not to get too frustrated when things don't go as planned.

One night, we thought we'd finally figured out our son's sleep schedule—only to have him stay up all night. Every time we got him down, he woke back up 15 minutes later. Was it frustrating? Absolutely. But over time, you learn to laugh at the unpredictability of it all and accept that this is just part of the adventure.

The Importance of Teamwork and Understanding

You and your partner are a team, and during the night shift, teamwork is essential. You'll have to rely on each other in ways you might not have before. One of the most important things we learned was the value of **understanding each other's struggles**. Sleep deprivation affects everyone differently, and it's easy to forget that your partner is going through it, too. When you're both running on fumes, patience can run thin, but that's when communication and empathy are most crucial.

There were times when my wife and I would snap at each other in the middle of the night. It's only natural when you're exhausted and dealing with a crying baby. But what got us through was the reminder that we were in it together. We'd apologize quickly, laugh about how ridiculous the situation was, and move on. It wasn't about who was doing more; it was about surviving as a team. Understanding that we were both doing our best, even when things felt overwhelming, made all the difference.

Finding the Humor in the Chaos

Here's a little secret: the night shift is going to be hard, but it's also going to be funny—eventually. Maybe not in the moment, but you'll look back on some of these sleepless nights and laugh. The delirium of sleep deprivation makes everything feel a little more absurd, and there's a kind of humor in how chaotic things get. Whether it's getting up for the fourth time in one night, fumbling with a diaper in the dark, or accidentally spilling water all over yourself while trying to juggle the baby, you'll find moments that make you smile in hindsight.

One night, I was so tired that when I went to grab a bottle from the fridge, I somehow knocked over half the contents of the fridge, causing a small cascade of food to hit the floor. My wife and I were too tired to clean it up, so we just left it there until morning. By the time we woke up, we couldn't stop laughing at how ridiculous the situation was. Those moments of shared exhaustion and humor are what get you through.

Embracing the Night Shift

The night shift isn't something to be feared—it's just a phase, albeit a challenging one. You'll get through it, and you'll even learn to appreciate the quiet moments with your baby in the middle of the night. There's something almost magical about those early hours, when it's just you and your newborn, with the rest of the world fast asleep.

As hard as it is, the night shift is an important part of fatherhood. It's when you really get to bond with your baby, in the stillness and quiet of the night. And once you get past the initial exhaustion, you'll start to see it as a unique, albeit exhausting, part of the journey.

Looking back, some of my favorite memories from those early days are from the middle of the night. Sure, I was tired, but there was something about holding our son in the dark, with just the soft hum of the white noise machine in the background, that felt special. Those moments, when it was just the two of us, are memories I wouldn't trade for anything.

So, fathers, remember this: you're stronger than you think, and you'll survive the night shift—one coffee-fueled diaper change at a time.

The minute you step into fatherhood, something fundamental shifts in your life. Suddenly, the priorities that once revolved around your career, hobbies, and personal goals take a backseat to a much bigger responsibility—being a dad. And while it's an incredible, life-changing experience, balancing work life and fatherhood can feel like trying to juggle flaming swords while riding a unicycle. The good news? You can adapt without burning out. It's all about time management, understanding your limits, and setting realistic expectations.

In this chapter, we're going to dive into what it really means to juggle a career and fatherhood, provide tips for creating a work-life balance that works for you, and, of course, sprinkle in a bit of humor along the way.

---

1. The Reality Check: Expect Things to Get Messy

The first thing you need to know about balancing work and fatherhood is that *balance* is a loose term. Forget the idea that there's some perfect harmony where your baby, your job, and your personal time all align flawlessly. You're going to have days where everything feels like it's falling apart, and other days where it all somehow clicks into place. The key is accepting that messiness is part of the process.

Here's a story from my own experience. When my son was born, I had just finished up working nights. I thought I was ready for the switch to fatherhood—I was already used to getting up early and handling unpredictable hours. But let me tell you, nothing quite prepares you for the sleep deprivation that comes with a newborn. You think pulling an all-nighter at work is tough? Try staying up with a crying baby who refuses to sleep, then heading into the office the next morning. It's like trying to solve a math problem while running on three brain cells and half a cup of coffee.

But here's the thing: it's possible. You adjust. You figure it out as you go, and you learn to give yourself grace when things don't go according to plan.

---

2. Prioritizing What Matters Most

Balancing work and fatherhood is about knowing what truly matters. The truth is, not everything deserves your immediate attention, and not everything is going to be perfect. You've got to learn to prioritize.

At work, focus on the tasks that drive results. Maybe this means cutting down on unnecessary meetings or finding ways to be more efficient with your time. For me, this meant mastering the art of *delegation*. If you have a team, learn to trust them with the small stuff so you can focus on what's important. The same goes for home life—don't stress about having the house spotless every day. Believe me, with a baby in the picture, it's not going to happen. Prioritize spending time with your child and being present for your partner.

---

3. Setting Boundaries at Work and at Home

A lot of dads, myself included, struggle with setting boundaries—especially when it comes to work. We want to be the best providers, which sometimes means overcommitting to long hours or bringing work home. But one of the biggest lessons I've learned is that setting clear boundaries at work helps you be a better dad at home.

It might be tough but start by having an honest conversation with your boss or colleagues. Let them know you're committed to your job, but you've also got a family that needs your attention. Set expectations around when you're available, and more importantly, when you're *not*. For example, if you're in the habit of answering emails late at night, try unplugging after a certain time so you can fully focus on family time.

Similarly, set boundaries at home. It's okay to carve out a little personal time—whether it's going to the gym, reading, or just having a moment to yourself. It helps keep you grounded and less likely to feel overwhelmed. You can't pour from an empty cup, and taking care of yourself ensures you're better equipped to take care of your family.

---

4. The Art of Flexibility: Adapting to the Chaos

Being flexible is a huge part of balancing work and fatherhood. Babies don't follow schedules, and as much as you plan, life will throw you curveballs. If you go into fatherhood expecting to control every aspect of your day, you're in for a rude awakening. Learning to adapt to chaos without losing your mind is key.

For instance, I've had days where I thought I had everything mapped out—work from 9 to 5, come home, handle bath time, get the baby to bed, and then maybe, just maybe, squeeze in a workout. Instead, I'd get a call from daycare saying my son was sick, and the whole day's plan would unravel. But it's in those moments you learn the value of flexibility.

If you're a rigid planner like me, this will take some practice, but try to leave room for the unexpected. You might not finish that project today, or you might have to reschedule that meeting to take care of your little one. That's okay. Your boss, your team, and your clients will understand. And when they don't? Well, that's what PTO and family leave are for.

---

5. Teamwork Makes the Dream Work

If you're in a relationship, balancing work and fatherhood is a team sport. You and your partner are going to have to communicate more than ever before—and not just about the baby's feeding schedule. Talk about how you're both feeling, what's stressing you out, and how you can support each other.

For my wife and me, teamwork was essential. We rotated duties, from nighttime feedings to diaper changes, and it made the load lighter for both of us. If I had an important meeting the next morning, she'd take on more of the night shifts. When she needed to catch up on sleep, I'd handle the baby for a few hours. It wasn't always a perfect system, but it worked for us because we were open about what we needed from each other.

If you're a single dad, teamwork doesn't just have to involve a partner. Lean on your support system—whether it's family, friends, or even a close co-worker. You'd be surprised how many people are willing to lend a hand if you ask.

---

6. The Importance of Self-Care: Avoiding Burnout

Here's the part where I get real with you. Burnout is a very real thing, especially for new dads trying to juggle it all. Between work, baby duties, and trying to maintain some semblance of your previous life, it's easy to neglect yourself. But here's the kicker: you can't take care of others if you don't take care of yourself.

Whether it's finding time for a hobby, getting back into the gym, or simply taking a nap when the baby naps, self-care is crucial. You'll be a better dad and a better employee if you're not running on fumes.

For me, working nights was a bit of a blessing in disguise when it came to avoiding burnout. I was already used to the strange hours and lack of sleep, so transitioning into paternity leave didn't hit me as hard as I thought it would. But even so, I still had to make time to rest and recharge—whether that meant going for a quick run in the morning or watching a show with my wife in the evening.

The key is finding balance in the imbalance. Some weeks you'll feel like you're nailing it at work but struggling at home, and other weeks it'll be the opposite. But if you carve out moments to take care of yourself, it'll all feel a lot more manageable.

---

7. Embrace the New Normal

Finally, understand that fatherhood changes you—and that's not a bad thing. Your career is still important, but it's no longer the center of your universe. Your priorities have shifted, and while that can be intimidating, it's also deeply fulfilling.

Instead of fighting the changes that fatherhood brings, embrace them. Recognize that it's okay to say no to an extra project at work if it means spending more time with your baby. Accept that you might not be able to hang out with your buddies as often, or that your workout routine might need to change. Life as you knew it is different now, but different doesn't mean worse—it just means you're adapting to a new chapter.

And if you're feeling overwhelmed by the balancing act, remember this: nobody has it all figured out. Every dad struggles with the same questions and challenges. The important thing is to keep showing up, keep communicating, and keep trying your best.

Conclusion: You've Got This

Balancing work life and fatherhood is a challenge, no doubt about it. But with a little flexibility, a lot of communication, and a good dose of humor, you'll find your groove. You won't always get it right—and that's okay. But you'll learn, you'll adapt, and you'll keep moving forward.

So, to the soon-to-be dad reading this, take a deep breath. You're stepping into the greatest, messiest, and most rewarding role of your life. And no matter how many sleepless nights or chaotic workdays are ahead, remember: you've got this.

Chapter 9

Dodging the Dad-Bod—Finding Time to Stay Fit as a New Dad

Ah, the "dadbod"—the mythical creature that sneaks up on you when you least expect it. One minute you're in decent shape, hitting the gym regularly, feeling good about yourself, and then BAM! The sleepless nights, extra stress, and convenient take-out meals start piling up, and suddenly you've got a little extra padding around the midsection. Welcome to fatherhood.

But here's the good news: you don't have to let the dadbod win. While it's easy to fall into the trap of letting your fitness slide, it's just as easy to make sure you stay on track, even if you're juggling diaper changes, sleepless nights, and a crying baby. You don't need hours at the gym or complex routines. What you need is a plan, some determination, and a little creativity.

So, let's talk about how to fit fitness into your life as a new dad. It's possible and trust me— you'll feel a hundred times better for it. Whether you've got five minutes or thirty, I've got you covered. Let's turn this "dadbod" into a "dad-who-is-fit-and-strong-bod."

The Dad Bod Dilemma

Let's start by addressing the elephant (or, rather, the donut) in the room: the dadbod. It's easy to see how it happens. You've got less time, more responsibilities, and your priorities shift. Suddenly, working out feels like a luxury, and the idea of hitting the gym seems like something from a past life. But here's the truth: staying fit as a dad isn't just about vanity— it's about being healthy, energized, and able to keep up with your kids as they grow.

The dadbod sneaks up on you because of **three key factors**:

1. **Lack of Time:** Babies are a time-suck. Between feedings, diaper changes, and trying to grab a few hours of sleep, finding time to work out seems impossible.
2. **Convenient (But Unhealthy) Food Choices:** When you're exhausted, it's tempting to reach for the quickest, easiest meal, and those meals aren't always the healthiest.
3. **Sleep Deprivation:** Let's be honest, sleep becomes a luxury when you have a newborn. And when you're tired, motivation to work out is low, and stress hormones like cortisol can lead to weight gain.

But here's the thing—if you make small, consistent efforts, you can still stay in shape. You just need to approach fitness differently than you did before becoming a dad.

Why Fitness Matters (Especially as a dad)

First things first—fitness isn't just about looking good in the mirror (though that's a nice bonus). Staying fit is about having the **energy** to keep up with your little ones, the **strength** to carry them around (because trust me, those car seats get heavy), and the **mental clarity** to deal with the ups and downs of fatherhood. Exercise reduces stress, boosts your mood, and helps you sleep better—everything you need to be the best dad you can be.

Plus, let's be real—your kids are watching you. You want to set a good example for them, showing them that taking care of your body is important, no matter how busy life gets.

I'll admit, after our son was born, I struggled with finding time to work out. The sleepless nights took a toll and squeezing in gym time felt like a pipe dream. But once I started making fitness a priority—even if it was just for 20 minutes here and there—I felt like a different person. More energized, less stressed, and honestly, just more capable of handling the chaos of fatherhood.

Finding Time for Fitness: The Dad-Friendly Approach

Now, here's the question every new dad asks: **"How can I find time to work out when I'm already so busy?"** The answer is simple: you've got to work smarter, not harder. Here's how:

---

1. Embrace Short, Efficient Workouts

Gone are the days when you could spend two hours at the gym. But guess what? You don't need that much time. In fact, **short, high-intensity workouts** can be just as effective (if not more so) than long gym sessions. You can get a great workout in 20-30 minutes if you focus on compound movements (think squats, push-ups, and deadlifts) that work multiple muscles at once.

During paternity leave, I'd sneak in a quick workout whenever I had 20 minutes. It wasn't about working out every day but making the most of the time I had. A quick 15-minute bodyweight circuit while the baby napped or a few sets of push-ups while waiting for dinner to cook—those short bursts of exercise add up.

---

2. Workout at Home (No Gym Required)

Let's face it—getting to the gym might not be realistic in the early days of fatherhood. But that doesn't mean you can't get a solid workout in at home. Bodyweight exercises like squats, push-ups, planks, and lunges require zero equipment and can be done right in your living room. If you want to level up, invest in a few dumbbells or resistance bands, which are affordable and easy to store.

Here's a simple, equipment-free routine that you can do anywhere:

- **Push-ups:** 3 sets of 12-15 reps
- **Squats:** 3 sets of 15-20 reps
- **Planks:** Hold for 30-60 seconds (3 sets)
- **Lunges:** 3 sets of 12-15 reps per leg

This takes less than 20 minutes but works your entire body. And the best part? You don't need to leave the house.

---

3. Turn Family Time into Fitness Time

Who says workouts must be solo? Get your family involved! Strap the baby into the stroller and go for a walk or a jog. If your child is old enough, turn playtime into a mini workout—lifting them up for a few reps or chasing them around the yard can get your heart rate up.

One of my favorite ways to get moving was by taking my son for a walk around the neighborhood. Pushing the stroller not only got me out of the house but also doubled as a cardio session. Plus, it was a great way to bond with him while giving my wife a break.

---

4. Prioritize Your Workouts

You must treat your workouts like an essential part of your day—because they are. Schedule them like appointments, even if it's just 15 minutes. Make them a non-negotiable part of your routine. It might mean waking up 20 minutes earlier or squeezing in a quick workout during your lunch break, but trust me, it's worth it.

I learned quickly that if I didn't plan my workouts, they wouldn't happen. So, I made a point to schedule them into my day. Sometimes that meant a quick workout before the baby woke up in the morning, other times it was during his nap. Having a plan made all the difference.

---

5. Make Nutrition Simple and Sustainable

Working out is only half the battle—what you eat plays a huge role in how you feel and look. As a dad, you'll need **quick, healthy meals** that fit into your busy schedule. Focus on whole foods like lean protein, veggies, fruits, and whole grains. And no, you don't need to follow some super strict diet. Just aim for balance and consistency.

Meal prep became my secret weapon. On Sundays, I'd cook up a bunch of chicken, rice, and veggies so that during the week, I had quick, healthy meals ready to go. It made it easier to stay on track and avoid the temptation of ordering takeout every night.

The Power of Consistency

Here's the secret to beating the dadbod: **consistency**. You don't need to be perfect, and you don't need to work out every day. What you do need is to make fitness a regular part of your routine. Even if it's just 10 minutes here and there, those small efforts will add up over time.

There were weeks when I only managed to work out twice, and other weeks when I could squeeze in four sessions. The key was to keep showing up, even when I didn't feel like it. It wasn't about going all out every time, but about being consistent.

Finding Motivation When You're Exhausted

Let's be real—there are going to be days when you're so tired that the idea of working out feels impossible. And that's okay. Some days, rest is more important than pushing yourself. But on the days when you can, remember that even a little bit of movement is better than nothing.

There were mornings when I felt like a zombie after being up half the night with our son. On those days, I'd go for a walk instead of doing a full workout. It wasn't about perfection—it was about moving my body and doing what I could.

Your Dad Bod, Your Rules

At the end of the day, fitness as a dad isn't about six-pack abs or hitting personal records in the gym. It's about staying healthy, feeling good, and having the energy to show up for your family. Whether that means a daily 20-minute workout or just finding time to stretch and move, it's all about balance. Remember that being a dad isn't a sprint, it's a marathon. Your fitness routine has to fit into your new life, not compete with it.

If you miss a workout or have a day where it feels like all you did was bounce a baby and chug coffee, **don't sweat it**—pun intended. Consistency doesn't mean perfection. What matters is that you keep trying, keep moving, and keep doing your best. The goal isn't to be shredded; it's to be **fit enough** to feel great, to keep up with your kids, and to be there for the long haul.

Practical Workout Plans for New Dads

Let's get into some practical ways to stay fit without feeling like it's one more overwhelming task on your plate. The key is to **simplify your fitness routine** and make it something you can actually stick to, no matter how crazy life gets. Here are some fitness plans that fit into a dad's busy schedule:

1. The 15-Minute Dad-Body Burner (No Equipment Needed)

If you only have a few minutes, this bodyweight circuit will get the job done. You can do this at home, no gym required. Here's how it works:

- **Squats (Bodyweight):** 3 sets of 20 reps
- **Push-Ups:** 3 sets of 15 reps
- **Plank:** Hold for 30-60 seconds (3 times)
- **Jumping Jacks:** 3 sets of 30 seconds
- **Mountain Climbers:** 3 sets of 20 reps (each side)

This whole routine takes about 15 minutes, but it gets your heart rate up and hits all the major muscle groups. It's perfect when the baby's napping, and you've got just a little window of time. Pro tip: set your timer and **don't stop** until it's done!

2. The 30-Minute Power Dad Workout (Minimal Equipment)

If you've got a little more time or want to invest in some dumbbells or resistance bands, this 30-minute routine will give you a more intense workout.

- **Dumbbell Squats:** 3 sets of 12-15 reps
- **Push-Ups or Dumbbell Bench Press:** 3 sets of 15 reps
- **Bent-Over Rows (with dumbbells):** 3 sets of 12-15 reps
- **Lunges:** 3 sets of 10 reps (each leg)
- **Plank:** Hold for 60 seconds
- **Burpees (for cardio):** 3 sets of 10 reps

This workout packs a punch but still fits into a 30-minute window. And let's face it, after 30 minutes, you're probably going to get interrupted by the baby waking up, so make the most of the time you've got!

3. "Baby on Board" Cardio

Sometimes, your baby is your workout buddy. One of the easiest ways to get moving is to **turn stroller walks into cardio sessions**. Walking is underrated, and pushing that stroller adds some extra resistance. Pop on a podcast or some music and turn a leisurely stroll into a power walk. It's a great way to get some fresh air, give your partner a break, and squeeze in some low-impact cardio. Bonus: fresh air might just get the baby to nap longer!

Balancing Fatherhood and Fitness

One of the biggest challenges dads face is **balancing time**—and fitness is often the first thing to fall by the wayside. But, as we've discussed, it doesn't have to be an all-or-nothing game. Small, consistent actions are better than sporadic, intense efforts.

Here's a reminder: the dadbod is just a label. There's no rule that says fatherhood automatically comes with extra weight or less fitness. You're in control of how you approach your health, and while you might not have as much time as you once did, you **can** still stay fit. Remember, even the smallest effort is a step in the right direction.

After our son was born, I felt overwhelmed at times. The pressure of getting everything right as a new dad, helping my wife, and trying to stay in shape felt like juggling a dozen things at once. But once I let go of the idea that I had to hit the gym for an hour every day or follow some strict routine, it became easier. I worked out when I could, and I didn't stress when I couldn't. That mindset shift made all the difference.

Tips for Staying Consistent as a Busy Dad

Let's wrap this up with some practical tips to help you stay consistent with your fitness goals:

---

1. Plan Ahead

If you don't schedule your workouts, they won't happen. Treat them like important meetings—put them in your calendar and stick to them. Whether it's a quick session during the baby's nap or a morning run before the chaos starts, having a plan makes all the difference.

---

2. Be Flexible

Life as a dad is unpredictable, so don't beat yourself up if things don't go according to plan. Missed your workout today? No worries. Jump back in tomorrow. The key is to stay flexible and adapt to your new reality.

3. Prioritize Sleep (Seriously)

We all know sleep is a rare commodity as a new parent, but you need to prioritize it as much as possible. When you're sleep-deprived, everything else becomes harder—including working out. If you're exhausted, rest. Your body needs it. But when you've gotten a decent night's sleep (or at least a decent nap), seize the opportunity to move.

4. Make Fitness Fun

If you hate working out, you won't stick to it. Find something you enjoy, whether it's a home workout, a jog, or even chasing your kids around the yard. The more fun it is, the more likely you'll keep doing it.

5. Celebrate Small Wins

It's easy to get discouraged if you're not seeing big changes but remember that progress is progress. Did you squeeze in a 10-minute workout today? Awesome. Managed to avoid the fast-food drive-thru? Good for you. Celebrate the small wins—they add up.

The Takeaway

Fatherhood is a journey that challenges you in ways you never imagined. Staying fit while raising kids isn't always easy, but it's possible. And you don't have to choose between being a great dad and taking care of yourself—you can do both. The key is finding balance, being consistent, and cutting yourself some slack when things don't go perfectly.

So, here's the deal: don't let the dadbod become your default. It's easy to fall into that trap, but it's just as easy to pull yourself out of it with a little determination, some creativity, and a lot of flexibility. You've got this.

Now, drop and give me 20 push-ups... or, you know, go change a diaper. Either way, you're doing great, Dad. Keep it up.

And with that, we've rounded off our deep dive into the "dadbod dilemma" and how to overcome it. You're stronger than you think, and staying fit as a dad is totally doable—even if it feels like chaos at times.

Ah, baby milestones—those precious moments that make all the sleepless nights, diaper blowouts, and endless feedings worth it. Whether it's their first smile, their first steps, or the first time they say "dada" (which, yes, *should* happen before "mama," but we'll get to that), watching your child hit these little life events is both exhilarating and, at times, terrifying.

Milestones are like those checkpoints in video games. Just when you think you've got things under control, bam! A new skill unlocks, and you're off to the next challenge. The best part? You'll find yourself cheering for the smallest things—because to your baby, they're huge.

In this chapter, we'll cover the major milestones you can expect in your child's early years, from birth up until around age 4. I'll break it down into different stages, so you know what to look forward to (and how to handle the overwhelming emotions that come with it).

---

0 to 6 Months: Welcome to the World!

The first six months are a whirlwind. One day, your baby is a tiny, wrinkly bundle of joy, and before you know it, they're giggling, rolling over, and grabbing at anything within reach—including your hair. Here are the milestones you can expect during this stage:

1. **Smiling (Around 6-8 Weeks)**
   That first real smile? Get ready, because it's going to melt your heart. And no, I'm not talking about those random, gas-induced grins they give in their sleep. I mean the *real* smile—when they look right at you and light up like you're the most amazing thing in the world. It usually happens between 6 to 8 weeks, and trust me, it'll make all those sleepless nights fade into the background.
2. **Lifting Their Head (Around 2-3 Months)**
   Around this time, your baby will start gaining neck strength and will be able to lift their head when they're on their tummy. It's like they're saying, "Hey, I'm not just a blob anymore—I can *move!*" It's also the moment when tummy time really starts to pay off, so if you've been struggling with getting them to do it, hang in there.
3. **Rolling Over (Around 4-6 Months)**
   Rolling over is a huge milestone. One day, they're just lying there, and the next day— boom! They're flipping over like an acrobat. This usually happens between 4 to 6 months, and once they figure it out, they'll keep doing it. So, if you thought changing diapers was tricky before, wait until your baby starts rolling mid-change. You'll need the reflexes of a ninja.
4. **Grabbing Things (Around 3-4 Months)**
   By this age, your baby's little hands will start reaching for things, which is adorable until they grab your coffee mug and send it flying. But it's all part of their development, and it's a sign that they're learning to interact with the world. Be

prepared to baby-proof your home, though, because once they can grab, everything becomes fair game.

---

6 to 12 Months: The Explorer Phase

By this stage, your baby has transitioned from a tiny newborn to a mini-explorer. Everything is new, exciting, and absolutely needs to be put in their mouth. Here's what to expect during this phase:

1. **Sitting Up (Around 6-8 Months)**
   Sitting up is a game-changer. Once your baby can sit on their own, they have a whole new perspective on the world. It usually happens between 6 to 8 months, and while it might seem like a small thing, it's actually a huge step in their development. It's also the stage where you can finally plop them in front of some toys and not have to worry (too much) about them toppling over.
2. **Crawling (Around 7-10 Months)**
   When babies learn to crawl, nothing is safe. You'll blink, and suddenly, they're halfway across the room, headed straight for that electrical outlet you forgot to cover. Crawling typically happens between 7 to 10 months, and it's their first real taste of independence. It's also when your job gets a whole lot harder because you'll be chasing them everywhere.
3. **Pulling Up to Stand (Around 9-12 Months)**
   Around 9 to 12 months, your baby will start pulling themselves up to stand. It's like they've decided, "Okay, crawling is fun, but walking? That's the next level." Once they start pulling up, it won't be long before they're cruising around the furniture and eyeing the stairs with an evil glint in their eye.
4. **First Words (Around 9-12 Months)**
   The moment you've been waiting for—your baby's first word. It'll probably be something like "dada," "mama," or, if you're really lucky, "no." This typically happens between 9 to 12 months, and it's one of the most exciting milestones. If they say "dada" first, you get to lord it over your partner (for a little while, at least).

---

12 to 24 Months: Walking and Talking (aka the Toddler Tornado)

Once your baby hits their first birthday, things really start ramping up. They're walking, they're talking (sort of), and they're getting into everything. Here's what to expect in the toddler phase:

1. **Walking (Around 12-15 Months)**
   Those wobbly first steps are one of the biggest milestones of all. It usually happens around 12 to 15 months, and once they're up on two feet, there's no turning back.

Watching your child take their first steps is both thrilling and terrifying because you realize that your days of sitting peacefully are officially over.

2. **Saying More Words (Around 18-24 Months)**
   By this age, your toddler's vocabulary will start expanding. They'll go from saying one or two words to stringing together simple sentences. "No, Daddy!" and "Mine!" will become common phrases, but don't worry—they'll also start saying cute things like "I love you," which totally makes up for the sass.

3. **Climbing Everything (Around 18-24 Months)**
   If there's something to climb, your toddler will find it. Chairs, couches, bookshelves—nothing is off-limits. This newfound love of climbing can be a bit nerve-wracking, but it's all part of their development. Just make sure you've got plenty of pillows nearby for soft landings.

4. **Pretend Play (Around 18-24 Months)**
   Around this age, your toddler will start engaging in pretend play, which is both adorable and hilarious. They'll pretend to cook, drive a car, or take care of their stuffed animals. It's a sign that their imagination is developing, and it's also a great way to bond with them.

---

2 to 4 Years: The Little Human Emerges

By the time your child hits age 2, they've officially entered "little human" territory. They're walking, talking, and showing off their personality in full force. Here's what to expect from the toddler-to-preschooler transition:

1. **Running and Jumping (Around 2-3 Years)**
   At this stage, your child will not only be walking, but running—and they'll run *everywhere*. They'll also start jumping, climbing, and generally testing the limits of their physical abilities. It's like they've discovered a new gear, and they're determined to use it at full speed.

2. **Speaking in Full Sentences (Around 3-4 Years)**
   By age 3 to 4, your child will be speaking in full sentences, and they'll have a lot to say. Sometimes, it's sweet. Other times, it's hilarious. And occasionally, they'll hit you with a brutally honest truth you weren't prepared for. ("Daddy, why is your tummy so big?")

3. **Playing with Others (Around 3-4 Years)**
   Around age 3 to 4, your child will start playing with other kids instead of just next to them. This is when you'll really see their social skills develop, and it's also the time when you'll start hearing all about their new "best friend" from preschool.

4. **Learning Colors, Shapes, and Numbers (Around 2-4 Years)**
   This is also the stage where your child will start learning the basics—colors, shapes, numbers, and even the alphabet. It's amazing to watch them soak up information like a sponge, and before you know it, they'll be showing off their newfound knowledge to anyone who will listen.

Cherish Every Moment

The milestones your child hits in these first four years are truly incredible to witness. They grow so fast, and every new skill they develop feels like a mini miracle. But here's the thing—there's no need to stress about hitting every milestone right on time. Babies develop at their own pace, and as long as they're moving forward, you're doing great.

Every first smile, step, and word is a moment you'll never forget. And while it might feel overwhelming at times, try to take a step back and appreciate these milestones as they happen. After all, these early years fly by faster than you can imagine.

Chapter 11

Dad and Baby Bonding: Building That Unbreakable Connection

Bonding with your baby as a new dad is one of the most rewarding parts of fatherhood. While you may not have carried them for nine months or experienced the emotional roller coaster of pregnancy, your connection with your little one is just as essential and powerful. Creating that bond can feel a bit overwhelming at first—after all, newborns don't exactly come with an instruction manual (wouldn't that be nice, though?).

But here's the good news: there are plenty of ways to bond with your baby that feel natural and enjoyable, whether you're a hands-on dad or just figuring things out. Some dads feel a strong connection immediately, while others take a little more time to find their groove. Either way, you're building a foundation that will last a lifetime.

In this chapter, we'll dive into practical ways for dads to bond with their babies, from skin-to-skin contact to those everyday moments that strengthen your relationship. Let's get into it.

---

1. Skin-to-Skin: The First Bonding Experience

I'll start with one of the most powerful bonding experiences: *skin-to-skin contact*. This method is often suggested right after birth, and I can tell you from personal experience—it's a game-changer. When my son was born, I used skin-to-skin contact to help calm him down, and it worked like magic. Holding your baby against your chest, feeling their tiny heartbeat next to yours, creates an immediate sense of security for them and a deep connection for you.

Here's why it's so effective:

- It helps regulate your baby's body temperature, heart rate, and breathing.
- It boosts oxytocin (the bonding hormone) for both you and the baby.
- It can reduce stress for the baby and helps them feel comforted.

So, if you get the chance, ditch the shirt, and let your baby snuggle up on your chest. Those moments are priceless, and they'll create a bond you won't forget.

2. The Art of Feeding Time: Bottle Bonding

If your partner is breastfeeding, it's easy to feel like you're on the sidelines. But feeding time is one of the best opportunities for dads to bond, especially if you're bottle-feeding or handling expressed milk.

When I fed my son, I took it as a chance to slow down, hold him close, and make it a special dad-and-baby moment. You'll find that, even in the midst of all the chaos, feeding time can become one of the most peaceful parts of your day (or night).

To make feeding time even more bonding:

- Hold your baby close to your chest, look into their eyes, and talk to them softly.
- Sing to them if you're feeling up to it—even if you're completely tone-deaf, they won't mind!
- Make sure you're calm and present, especially during night feeds. These small moments add up.

3. Diaper Duty: Surprisingly, a Great Bonding Opportunity

Let's be honest: no one *enjoys* changing diapers. It's not glamorous, but it's a necessity, and guess what? It's also an excellent bonding opportunity.

For me, changing diapers was brand-new territory, and I had no idea what I was doing at first. But after a few changes, I realized it wasn't just about getting through the dirty work. It was a chance to care for my son in a way that was intimate, attentive, and, yes, even loving. The key is to approach diaper duty not as a chore, but as a time to interact and connect.

Make it a bonding experience by:

- Talking or singing to your baby while you change them. It helps distract them and makes the process smoother.
- Using the time to engage in gentle play—tickling their toes or making funny faces can keep things light.
- Not rushing it. Sure, you want to get it done, but slow down and use those moments to engage.

4. Bedtime Routines: A Daily Ritual for Bonding

One of the most consistent ways to bond with your baby is through a bedtime routine. Babies and toddlers thrive on routines—they make them feel safe and secure. And for dads, it's a chance to create a special moment every day that's just for the two of you.

When I helped put my son to bed, I made it a calming experience. Whether it was reading a story, giving him a bath, or singing (even badly), it became part of our ritual. These small moments, done consistently, build a bond over time.

Here's how to create a bedtime bonding routine:

- **Bath time**: If your baby loves the water, bath time can be a great bonding experience. Use the time to play, splash around, and enjoy some relaxed moments together.
- **Storytime**: Even if your baby is too young to understand words, reading to them at night is a great way to introduce language and soothe them with your voice. Plus, it's a tradition you can keep up as they grow.
- **Cuddles and calm**: After the bath and story, cuddle up and spend a few minutes just holding them close before bed. It's a perfect way to end the day on a connected note.

---

5. Getting Active: Bonding Through Movement

As your baby grows, they'll become more active, and so will you. One of the best ways to bond with them is by getting involved in their movement and play. Whether it's tummy time, rolling over, crawling, or those first wobbly steps, being right there with them creates a deep connection.

I loved getting on the floor with my son and playing during his tummy time. Watching him struggle to push up or try to roll over wasn't just cute—it was a way to cheer him on and be part of his physical development.

Ways to bond through movement:

- **Tummy time**: Get down on the floor with them and make funny faces, sounds, or hold toys to encourage them. Tummy time is great for their muscle development and is even better with dad cheering them on.
- **Active play**: As your baby becomes more mobile, engage in active play like crawling together, rolling around, or using baby toys that involve interaction.
- **Helping with milestones**: Be present during big moments like first steps or learning to stand. Your involvement in these physical milestones will help them feel supported and loved.

---

6. Talking and Communicating: The Power of Your Voice

From the moment your baby is born, they're soaking up everything around them—including your voice. Talking to your baby is one of the easiest and most effective ways to bond. And no, it doesn't matter if they don't understand the words yet. Babies pick up on tone, rhythm, and the sound of your voice, all of which help them feel connected to you.

When I started talking to my son, I felt a little silly at first—after all, I was just narrating my day to a tiny human who had no idea what I was saying. But over time, I noticed that he responded more to my voice, and it became one of our ways to connect.

To make the most of talking and communication:

- **Narrate your day.** Whether you're making breakfast or driving to the store, talk to your baby about what's happening. It helps build language skills and makes them feel engaged.
- **Sing.** I know I've mentioned it a few times, but even if you're not a great singer, babies love the sound of their parent's voice. Create silly songs or sing lullabies—it all strengthens your bond.
- **Respond to their sounds.** As your baby starts making cooing or babbling sounds, respond like you're having a real conversation. It shows them you're listening and encourages them to keep communicating.

---

7. Going on Adventures: Exploring the World Together

One of the most fun ways to bond with your baby is by going on little adventures together. Whether it's a trip to the park, a walk around the neighborhood, or a day at the zoo, exploring the world through your baby's eyes is an incredible experience.

When my son was just a few months old, my wife and I took trips to get out of the house and clear our heads. Being outdoors and showing our son the beauty of nature (even though he probably didn't appreciate it at the time) was a special bonding experience. It's a reminder that bonding doesn't have to be complicated—sometimes, it's just about spending time together in new places.

To make adventures special:

- **Go on walks**: Put your baby in a carrier or stroller and go for walks. Fresh air and a change of scenery can do wonders for both you and the baby.
- **Explore new environments**: Take your baby to new places—parks, beaches, zoos. Seeing the world through their eyes makes even the simplest outings feel magical.
- **Make memories**: Bring a camera and take photos of your adventures. Even though your baby won't remember these trips, you'll have the memories to look back on.

---

8. Listening and Being Present: Quality Over Quantity

It's not always about how much time you spend with your baby—it's about the *quality* of that time. Whether you're working full-time or staying at home, being present during the moments you have with your child is what really counts.

For me, even though I worked nights, I made sure to make the most of the time I had with my son. Whether it was early mornings before I went to bed or during my days off, I focused on being fully present and engaged.

To be more present:

- **Put the phone down**: It's easy to get distracted by technology, but when you're with your baby, try to focus on them instead of checking your phone.
- **Engage with them**: Even when they're very young, babies pick up on whether you're engaged. Make eye contact, talk to them, and be part of their world.
- **Make the most of small moments**: Even if you don't have hours to spend with your baby every day, those little moments add up. A few minutes of focused play or cuddling can mean the world to your child.

Conclusion

Bonding with your baby is a lifelong journey, and it starts with those early moments when they're small and helpless. Whether it's through skin-to-skin contact, talking to them, or just being present during everyday routines, every dad has their own way of building that connection. Don't worry if it takes time—you're both learning and growing together.

The most important thing? Be there. Be present. And remember, every small effort you make to bond with your child lays the foundation for a relationship that will last a lifetime. Plus, these moments are precious—you'll look back on them someday and realize they were some of the best days of your life.

Chapter 12

Dad Fails and How to Fix Them: Embrace the Chaos and Learn Along the Way

No dad is perfect. Not even close. In fact, there are days where you might feel like you're winging it and others when it's clear you've flat-out dropped the ball (hopefully not the baby). Fatherhood is a learning experience, and if there's one universal truth, it's that every dad makes mistakes. The trick? Learn from them, adapt, and keep going. So, let's dive into some classic dad fails, laugh a little, and talk about how to turn those mistakes into lessons.

1. The "Forgot to Pack the Diaper Bag" Disaster

Scenario: You're about to head out with your baby for what seems like a quick trip to the grocery store. You're thinking, "It's just 20 minutes—do I really need to pack a full diaper bag?" You skip the essentials. Halfway through the trip, the baby decides it's time for a blowout of epic proportions, and you're standing there with nothing but your wallet and some grocery coupons.

The Mistake: Underestimating just how quickly things can go from peaceful to catastrophic when it comes to babies.

How to Fix It: Always—**always**—pack a diaper bag. Even for short trips, pack the essentials: diapers, wipes, a spare outfit, and a snack. Trust me, you'll thank yourself later. The one time you think, "I won't need it," will be the time you need it most. It's like the universe knows.

2. The "Overconfident Assembler" Debacle

Scenario: The new crib or highchair arrives, and you're ready to channel your inner handyman. The instructions? Pfft, who needs 'em? Thirty minutes later, you've got parts that don't fit, screws that mysteriously disappeared, and a structure that looks more like abstract art than a functional baby product.

The Mistake: Going full DIY without checking the instructions (or worse, checking them and ignoring them).

How to Fix It: As tempting as it is to flex your DIY muscles, always read the manual. And if you're not naturally gifted with a wrench, it's okay to ask for help. In fact, make it a team effort. You can assemble, and your partner can laugh at you when you try to shove part C into part A upside down. Bonus points if the baby watches, making you feel like you're already failing as a role model.

3. The "I Can Totally Handle This" Sleep Deprivation Episode

Scenario: You've been getting four hours of sleep a night for the last week, but today's the day you're going to prove you can still function like a normal adult. Coffee in hand, you start tackling the day. That's when things start to fall apart. You forget to put the laundry in the dryer, accidentally pour formula into your own coffee, and leave the house in two different shoes.

The Mistake: Overestimating how well you can function on little to no sleep.

How to Fix It: Sleep deprivation is a reality for most new parents, but that doesn't mean you should push through it like a hero. If you're exhausted, let someone else take over for a bit, even if it's just for a 20-minute power nap. And on those days where you're in zombie mode, give yourself grace. You're not going to be operating at 100%, and that's okay.

4. The "Public Tantrum" Panic

Scenario: You're out at a restaurant with your toddler, enjoying what you thought was a calm family meal. But the moment the food arrives, your little one decides now is the perfect time to throw a tantrum. It's loud. It's dramatic. And every head in the place is turning toward you.

The Mistake: Trying to reason with a toddler mid-meltdown. It's like negotiating with a tiny, irrational dictator.

How to Fix It: The first rule of public tantrums is don't panic. Take a deep breath and calmly remove your child from the situation if possible. Trying to reason or bribe them in the middle of a meltdown rarely works. And here's a secret: everyone around you has either been there or will be. Don't worry about what other people think—just focus on getting through it.

5. The "I Can Fix This" Emotional Shutdown

Scenario: Your partner is stressed. They've been home with the baby all day, and they're at their wit's end. You listen to them vent, and being the problem-solver that you are, you start offering solutions: "Why don't you try this?" or "Have you thought about doing it this way?"

The Mistake: Jumping into "fix it" mode when all your partner wanted was for you to listen.

How to Fix It: Sometimes, the best thing you can do is just be there and listen. Not everything requires a solution—sometimes, people just need to vent. Resist the urge to fix and instead offer support. A simple "I hear you" or "That sounds really tough" goes a long way.

6. The "Forgot the Car Seat" Fiasco

Scenario: You've been meticulously preparing for the big day: birth day. Bags are packed, snacks are ready, and you've memorized the quickest route to the hospital. Everything is perfect...except the car seat. It's still sitting in its box at home, and you didn't realize it until you're in the hospital, ready to bring the baby home.

The Mistake: Assuming you have more time than you actually do to handle the little details.

How to Fix It: Start early with things like setting up the car seat, babyproofing the house, and prepping the nursery. Babies have a way of arriving when they feel like it, not necessarily on your schedule. A little prep work goes a long way in reducing last-minute panic.

7. The "Underestimating the Mess" Mistake

Scenario: You're feeling confident. Your baby is freshly bathed, in a new outfit, and you're about to head out for a family event. Suddenly, you hear the dreaded sound—diaper blowout. There's poop *everywhere*. On the baby, the changing table, and somehow, even on your shirt.

The Mistake: Thinking you can avoid major messes, especially at the worst possible times.

How to Fix It: Accept that messes are a part of the journey. Always keep spare outfits for both the baby and yourself handy (because, yes, poop can and will find you). And remember, these are the stories you'll laugh about later—even if they're gross in the moment.

8. The "Letting Guilt Take Over" Moment

Scenario: You've had a long day, and the last thing you want to do is play pretend tea party with your toddler. But the guilt starts creeping in. "Shouldn't I be cherishing every moment? Shouldn't I want to spend every waking second with my kid?"

The Mistake: Allowing guilt to dictate your parenting choices.

How to Fix It: Parenthood is exhausting, and it's okay if you don't want to play *every* time your kid asks. You're allowed to be tired. You're allowed to take a break. What matters is that you're there when it counts. Your child won't remember every tea party, but they will remember the times you showed up when they really needed you.

9. The "Technology Overload" Dilemma

Scenario: It's been a long day, and the easiest way to get some peace and quiet is to hand your child a tablet or let them watch TV for a couple of hours. But then you start worrying— is too much screen time going to turn my kid into a zombie?

The Mistake: Feeling like you've failed because you use technology as a break.

How to Fix It: Screen time in moderation is okay. Don't beat yourself up for letting your kid watch cartoons so you can catch your breath. The key is balance—make sure there's plenty of non-screen activities to, but know that using technology to give yourself a break doesn't make you a bad parent. It makes you human.

10. The "Expecting Perfection" Trap

Scenario: You had this vision of what kind of dad you'd be—perfect, patient, always on top of things. But reality is messy. There are days you lose your temper, days you forget important things, and days where you feel like you're just getting by.

The Mistake: Setting unrealistic expectations for yourself as a father.

How to Fix It: Let go of the idea of perfection. You're going to make mistakes. Lots of them. What matters is that you learn from those mistakes, keep showing up, and do your best. Your kids don't need a perfect dad—they just need *you*.

Final Thoughts: Embrace the Imperfections

Every dad makes mistakes. It's inevitable. But those mistakes are how you learn and grow as a father. The key is to embrace the imperfections, laugh at the absurdity, and keep moving forward. Fatherhood is a messy, chaotic, wonderful adventure, and the sooner you accept that mistakes are part of the package, the more you'll be able to enjoy the ride.

So, here's the deal: when you add a tiny, unpredictable human into your life, everything changes. I don't mean just your sleep schedule or the amount of laundry (though those change drastically too). The dynamic between you and your partner takes a hit—sometimes small, sometimes earth-shattering. No one can really prepare you for it, because no two relationships are the same, and no two babies are the same either.

One minute, you're a team that crushes Netflix binges and spontaneous date nights; the next, you're tag-teaming diaper duty at 3 a.m., arguing over who gets the last bit of sleep, and both of you are wearing the same sweatpants for days on end. It's messy, it's exhausting, and it's beautiful in its own weird way. But if there's one thing that's absolutely crucial when it comes to surviving this shift, it's learning to adapt to the changes. Because trust me, the changes come fast and furious, and there's no hitting pause.

In this chapter, we'll take a deep dive into how a baby can throw a wrench into even the best relationships, and, more importantly, how to adjust to those changes. After all, it's not about being perfect—it's about working together for the good of your family.

---

1. The Shift: From Lovers to Co-Parents

Before the baby, you and your partner were two adults in a relationship, maybe even carefree at times. Sure, you probably had your fair share of disagreements, but things were (relatively) simple. Then, the baby arrives, and suddenly you're not just a couple anymore—you're co-parents.

What Changes:

- Intimacy can take a backseat. Between exhaustion and baby duties, you may find that romance feels more like a distant memory than a priority.
- Conversations shift from planning weekends away to debating the best brand of diapers. Your relationship gets consumed by baby logistics.
- The daily stress can turn minor annoyances into major blowouts. It's easy for tensions to rise when both of you are running on fumes.

How to Adapt:

- **Make time for each other.** Even if it's just 10 minutes before bed to check in, talk about something other than the baby, and reconnect.
- **Celebrate the small wins.** Maybe you both survived a particularly rough night, or one of you remembered to grab groceries on the way home—celebrate those little victories. It helps reinforce the sense that you're in this together.

- **Be patient.** Things won't always go smoothly, and it's important to give each other grace. Just because things are tough now doesn't mean they'll stay that way forever.

---

2. The Teamwork Test: Sharing the Load

One thing that really tests a relationship after having a baby is the workload. There's a lot to do—feedings, diaper changes, laundry, doctor's appointments—and it's easy for things to feel lopsided if one person feels like they're carrying more weight.

For my wife and me, it was all about teamwork. We didn't always get it right (I mean, who does?), but we made it work by rotating tasks and talking openly about what needed to be done.

What Changes:

- There's no longer time for "keeping score." This is the moment where both partners need to pitch in and help, no matter what their previous roles were.
- The mental load becomes a real thing. Sure, there's the physical work of parenting, but don't underestimate the mental work—remembering appointments, managing the baby's routine, and keeping track of milestones.
- The resentment creeps in when one person feels like they're shouldering more than their share of the load.

How to Adapt:

- **Communicate early and often.** One of the most important things my wife and I did was talk—about what needed to be done, who was doing what, and how we were feeling about it. If one person is feeling overwhelmed, it's essential to say so, before resentment builds.
- **Divide tasks based on strengths.** If one of you is better at calming the baby, and the other is more efficient at managing the household logistics, lean into those strengths. Parenting is not about doing everything equally; it's about working together in a way that makes sense.
- **Rotate when needed.** For us, rotating tasks helped keep things fair. One week I might be on diaper duty, the next I'd take the night shift. That way, no one feels stuck doing the same thing over and over.

---

3. The Stress Factor: Handling the Downs

Let's face it—when you're sleep-deprived, overworked, and stressed about keeping this tiny human alive, arguments happen. A lot. Even the best of relationships go through rough patches in the early days of parenthood.

What Changes:

- **Stress levels skyrocket.** Parenting is one of the most stressful things you'll ever do, and that stress has a way of creeping into your relationship. Arguments may flare up over things that, pre-baby, wouldn't have even been an issue.
- **Patience wears thin.** When you're both running on little sleep and stretched thin, it's easy to snap at each other over the smallest things.
- **Feeling disconnected.** Sometimes, the stress can make you feel like you and your partner are on different planets, even when you're in the same room.

How to Adapt:

- **Don't let small things fester.** If something is bothering you, bring it up calmly and directly. Little annoyances can grow into big problems if left unchecked.
- **Find outlets for stress.** Whether it's taking a break for a workout, getting out for a walk, or having a night out with friends, both of you need time to blow off steam.
- **Reconnect when you can.** Even if it's just for a few minutes after the baby is asleep, make time to talk or do something together. Small moments of connection help keep the relationship strong amidst the chaos.

---

4. Rediscovering Your New "Normal"

One of the toughest things about becoming parents is accepting that your life as a couple is going to look different now. And that's okay. The goal isn't to get back to how things were before the baby—the goal is to create a new normal that works for you as a family.

What Changes:

- Date nights are rare, and when they do happen, they look a little different (think takeout and a movie after the baby goes to bed).
- Conversations shift to include more about parenting, but that doesn't mean you stop talking about your interests, dreams, and goals.
- Spontaneity takes a backseat. Everything requires more planning, and that's okay. It just takes getting used to.

How to Adapt:

- **Redefine date night.** It's not about fancy dinners or grand gestures anymore. A good date night might just be sharing ice cream on the couch after the baby goes to bed. The point is to carve out time together, no matter how small.
- **Set new goals together.** Having a baby shifts your priorities, but it doesn't mean you stop dreaming. Talk about what you both want as individuals and as parents—whether it's travel, career goals, or personal milestones. Parenting is about evolving, not losing yourselves.

- **Appreciate the small moments.** That 10 minutes of quiet time after the baby falls asleep might not feel like much, but it's the little moments that help you stay connected as a couple.

---

5. It's Okay to Ask for Help

One thing a lot of new parents (dads especially) struggle with is asking for help. There's this unspoken idea that you should be able to do it all on your own. But let me tell you, that's a recipe for burnout.

What Changes:

- Parenting can feel isolating at times, especially if you don't have a lot of outside support. It's easy to feel like you're in it alone.
- The pressure to "have it all together" can lead to stress, anxiety, and feeling overwhelmed.

How to Adapt:

- **Lean on each other.** If one of you is struggling, it's okay to ask for help. My wife and I supported each other through the hardest times by simply being there and stepping in when the other needed a break.
- **Get outside help if needed.** Whether it's a family member, a babysitter, or a friend, don't hesitate to ask for help when you need it. You don't have to do everything on your own.
- **Be honest with yourself.** Parenting is hard, and it's okay to admit when you're feeling overwhelmed. Talk to your partner, seek advice from other parents, or even consult a professional if you need to.

---

6. Remember, You're Still a Team

At the end of the day, you and your partner are still a team. Sure, the dynamic has changed, and there will be bumps along the way, but you're in this together. And while things may feel different, they can also be stronger.

What Changes:

- Your roles within the relationship shift as you take on new responsibilities as parents.
- The focus becomes more about the baby, but that doesn't mean you stop being partners.

How to Adapt:

- **Keep communicating.** The most important thing my wife and I learned was to keep talking—about everything. Whether it's how tired we are or what our plans for the future are, staying connected through conversation helped us maintain a strong relationship.
- **Support each other.** There will be days when one of you feels like you can't go on, and that's when the other steps in. We always had each other's back, and that made all the difference.
- **Celebrate your wins.** Parenting is tough, but it's also incredibly rewarding. Make sure to celebrate the moments of success, no matter how small they seem.

In the end, having a baby changes your relationship, but it doesn't have to break it. It's all about adapting, supporting each other, and keeping the bigger picture in mind.

Well, here we are. You've made it through this entire book—through the ups and downs, the funny moments, the awkward scenarios, the dirty diapers, the sleepless nights, and now you're standing at the edge of something remarkable. You're about to be a dad. Maybe you're already there, deep in the trenches, or maybe you're still waiting for that first, life-changing cry in the delivery room. Either way, if you've stuck with me this long, you're in good shape.

Here's the thing: fatherhood is unpredictable, it's messy, and at times it'll test you in ways you never saw coming. But it's also one of the most rewarding experiences life can throw at you. By the time you're done with this whole dad gig, you'll have learned things you didn't even know you needed to learn. You'll have discovered parts of yourself you didn't know existed.

In this final chapter, I want to leave you with the kind of advice that I wish I had known before my son was born—those nuggets of wisdom that make you realize, "Oh yeah, I've got this." I want you to walk into fatherhood with a little less fear, a lot more confidence, and, most importantly, the ability to laugh at yourself along the way.

---

1. Expect the Unexpected (And Laugh When It Happens)

No matter how many books you read, how much you prepare, or how many parenting classes you attend, you're never going to feel 100% ready for everything fatherhood throws at you. And that's okay. The truth is no one really knows what they're doing.

Remember that moment when I spat coffee all over my wife during contractions? That's a prime example of the unexpected. Did I plan for it? Absolutely not. But it happened, and you just have to roll with it. You'll have plenty of moments like that—whether it's a diaper explosion at the worst possible time, or the baby's sudden decision to start screaming in a silent restaurant. It's all part of the adventure.

Key takeaway: Laugh when things go wrong. Because they will, and your ability to take it in stride will make all the difference.

---

2. Trust Yourself (You Know More Than You Think You Do)

Here's a little secret that most new dads don't realize: you're more prepared than you think. Sure, the thought of holding a newborn may terrify you at first (they're so small and fragile, right?), but trust me, once you get into it, your instincts kick in.

There's no magic formula to being a dad. You'll figure it out as you go. You'll learn the sounds of your baby's cries, you'll develop a sixth sense for when they're about to spit up, and you'll somehow manage to rock them to sleep at 2 a.m. while half-asleep yourself.

Key takeaway: Don't doubt yourself. You were built for this. You'll make mistakes (we all do), but you'll also surprise yourself with how much you actually know.

---

3. It's Okay to Feel Overwhelmed (Ask for Help When You Need It)

Fatherhood is one of the most rewarding experiences you'll ever have, but it's also one of the most exhausting. There will be times when you feel like you're completely out of your depth, and that's totally normal. I can't tell you how many nights I sat there thinking, "Am I really cut out for this?" Spoiler: I was, and so are you.

The important thing is to remember that it's okay to ask for help when you need it. Whether it's your partner, your family, or a friend, no one expects you to do this alone. In fact, you shouldn't do it alone. Fatherhood is a team effort, and leaning on others will make you a better dad in the long run.

Key takeaway: You don't have to be a superhero. It's okay to ask for help, and it doesn't make you any less of a dad to admit when you need a break.

---

4. The "Dad Bod" Is Optional (But Keeping Healthy Is Important)

We've talked a bit about the "dad bod" in a previous chapter, but let's touch on it one last time. While it's easy to let fitness slip to the bottom of your priority list when you're balancing a newborn, work, and life in general, don't forget to take care of yourself.

Not just for vanity's sake, but because your kid will eventually want to run around with you, climb on your back, and play. And trust me, you'll want the energy to keep up. Staying fit and healthy isn't just about looking good in photos; it's about being there, active and involved, in your child's life.

Key takeaway: You don't have to be a gym rat, but keep moving, stay active, and make time for your own health. Your kid will thank you for it.

---

5. Your Relationship Will Change (And That's Okay)

One of the biggest changes that fatherhood brings is the shift in your relationship with your partner. We've touched on this already, but it's worth reiterating here: things will change. Your focus will shift from just the two of you to this little person who needs constant attention.

That's not to say your relationship with your partner has to suffer—it doesn't. In fact, this new chapter can bring you closer if you both commit to supporting one another. My wife and I definitely had our moments of stress and tension (there's nothing quite like arguing over who's more tired), but we always came back to the fact that we were in this together.

Key takeaway: Make time for each other. Even if it's just a quick chat before bed or a shared laugh over something ridiculous the baby did, staying connected as a couple will make all the difference in your parenting journey.

---

6. Enjoy the Little Moments (Because They Pass Quickly)

Here's a piece of advice you'll hear over and over again: "Enjoy every moment, because they grow up fast." And as much as it sounds like a cliché, it's 100% true.

One day, you'll be holding this tiny, squirming baby in your arms, and the next, they'll be taking their first steps, saying their first words, and running around the house like a whirlwind. It happens faster than you can imagine, and while it's easy to get caught up in the chaos, try to take a step back every now and then to just soak it all in.

I'll never forget the first time my son smiled at me. I was beyond exhausted, hadn't slept in what felt like days, and suddenly, there it was—a big, toothless grin that melted away all the stress. Those are the moments that make it all worth it.

Key takeaway: The little moments—those seemingly mundane, everyday things—are the ones you'll cherish the most. Don't rush through them; savor them.

---

7. There's No Perfect Dad (Just a Dad Who's Trying His Best)

If there's one thing I want you to take away from this entire book, it's this: there is no such thing as a perfect dad. There will be days when you nail it and feel like you've got everything under control. And there will be days when you feel like you've dropped the ball completely. That's normal.

Fatherhood isn't about being perfect—it's about being present. It's about showing up, doing your best, and learning as you go. Your child doesn't need a flawless dad; they just need one who's there, who loves them, and who's willing to figure it out along the way.

Key takeaway: Give yourself grace. You're going to make mistakes, and that's okay. What matters is that you're there, trying your best, and loving your kid unconditionally.

---

8. You're Not Alone (There's a Whole Dad Squad Out There)

Finally, remember that you're not in this alone. As you've seen throughout this book, there's a whole world of dads out there going through the exact same things you are. Whether you join a dad group, connect with other fathers online, or just swap stories with friends, leaning on that community can be a game-changer.

There's strength in numbers and being part of a "dad squad" can help you navigate the challenges, laugh at the crazy moments, and celebrate the wins together.

Key takeaway: Connect with other dads. Share your experiences, learn from theirs, and support each other along the way.

Closing Thoughts: Welcome to the Club

And with that, we've reached the end. If you've made it this far, congratulations—you're ready for fatherhood. Or at least, as ready as anyone can be. The truth is, no matter how much advice you get, nothing will fully prepare you for the ride ahead. But you've got this. You're going to be a great dad, not because you're perfect, but because you care enough to try.

Fatherhood is messy, exhausting, challenging, and more than a little chaotic, but it's also filled with love, laughter, and moments that will take your breath away. So take a deep breath, embrace the chaos, and get ready for the wildest, most rewarding adventure of your life.

Welcome to the dad club—you're going to crush it.

Inspiration for the Journey Ahead: As you close this book, remember: the fact that you're here, reading this, shows that you're already on the right path. You care, you're learning, and you're going to be an awesome dad. Now go out there, embrace every moment, and most of all—have fun with it.

www.ingramcontent.com/pod-product-compliance
Lightning Source LLC
Chambersburg PA
CBHW061730250726
48657CB00002B/861